Advance Praise

"Whether it's a job that is killing you, or other daily life stressors, *I Love My Job, but It's Killing Me* is my kind of prescription to take back your health and your life. All too often we rely on Western medicine to fix what ails us. Lesley's journey from sickness back to health reminds us that we have the power within to heal. She is living proof and her book is just the inspiration a person needs to begin taking those first few baby steps to feeling great once more."

– Carrie Wallace
Owner of Yoga in the Center; Mill Creek, Washington

"Setting healthy limits and boundaries in all aspects of our lives is essential to living life more fully! Lesley was able to change her life significantly for the better. Lesley articulates how she made changes in a way others can understand, and take steps to make a difference in their lives too."

– Heidi Howard MA, LMHC, CDP

Lesley Moffat, true to her teaching roots, explains and presents the how-to's of turning your health and well-being around in a clear manner. No medical jargon. No shaming. Clear explanations with real-life examples. Remember your favorite teacher growing up? The unmistakable invitation to succeed you received? This is just like that – the invitation to succeed you got from your favorite teacher, but Lesley's lesson is much more than academics. A must-read for everyone looking to take better care of themselves.

Ro Berkley

"This is a good read for anyone whose profession has them interacting with young people; teachers, paraprofessionals, counselors, and so forth. We are all caregivers but can easily lose sight of caring for ourselves. Thank you, Lesley, for sharing your story and your advice for those of us in the same predicament or those who risk those perils."

– Sandy Rogers
Music teacher, Meridian School District

"Although I'm not a teacher, the lessons taught in Lesley's book can be applied to the field I work in. I am a 911 dispatcher and we deal with chronic stress fatigue and illness. I hope to be able to share this with my coworkers and supervisors. I believe the new habits and lifestyle choices I will be making will show as positive change in my life."

– Lisa Hendrichsen Bradley
Dispatcher – 911

I am not a teacher. I am the parent of two students lucky enough to be part of Lesley Moffat's band programs. I have watched with awe her transform from a dedicated but often sick band director, to the svelte, powerful and inspirational person who wrote this book. When I saw her at the start of the 2017 school year after a year without kids at her school, my mouth dropped. I asked her if she had spent the summer at Super Model Camp! That was how profound her transformation was. Yes, she was thinner, but she seemed taller and had a radiance I had not yet seen in her. With an "I'll have what she's having" excitement, I have been waiting for this book, because although I am not a teacher, I have my own brand of workaholic and serial pleasing tendencies that need to be tuned up and redirected towards self-care and optimal wellbeing. Bravo on the book! It is an easy read, and I will refer to it again and again. Thank you - I'm finally on my way!

Connie Baldwin
Mom of 2 Musical Teens, Entrepreneur,
Recovering Please-a-Holic

My Daughter is in Mrs. Moffat's Wind Ensemble class. She came home and told me about her book and figured it would be an interesting read. What I can say as a working mother and business professional the life lessons are applicable beyond the teaching world. I identified with many of the experiences/stories used throughout the book. Thanks for sharing this with the world!

Sharon L. Wierschke
Band Mom / Amazon Review 2/14/2019

Folks, this fabulous gem isn't just for teachers! It's for anyone who finds the harried pace of modern life overwhelming, and even crushing when buried beneath decades of keeping ones nose to the grindstone and putting everyone else's needs above your own. Lesley Moffat takes you on a journey into the daily life of a working woman, who must juggle a demanding career with marriage and children and boundaries and the havoc wrecked by the lack thereof, and shows you how to get to the other side of the craziness with with your health and sanity intact. She's a wonderful storyteller, and an even better teacher. Using her life, and the life of her dear friend who died of cancer, as well as her students, she makes you feel like she knows you, like she knows me, and truly GETS how consuming the overwhelm can be. Not only does she paint a picture you're sure to resonate with, but she gives you a map, a beautiful blueprint, to help you navigate through the mess. I HIGHLY recommend this wonderful book!

Cindy Cooley
Author – *Messy Bed, Messy Head*

She explains what I feel people live with every day of their lives but can't pinpoint the difficulties they are experiencing. She's a breath of fresh air, gives good insight on how to compartmentalize the issues you might be experiencing and give easy to understand ways of resolving those issues without it feeling like it an unreachable goal. I've seen her transformation and she's an amazing person and inspiration. Thank you for sharing your trials you've faced, you're a true hero to many.

Deanne Bodyfelt
Former Band Mom

The relatability of this book is unreal. The hands on exercises and self evaluations can be applied within the everyday ins and outs of the teaching world. I was stunned to be able to relate to this book so easily. Very refreshing read and one I would recommend to anyone who needs to feel like they are not alone.

K. Reed

Amazon Review 2/22/2019

This is a great read with plenty of well thought out advice for stressed out teachers. The author relates her path to wellness that is easily relatable and inspiring to follow. She provides hands on exercises and self-evaluation programs that really help to pinpoint areas individuals can tailor to their own specific needs. Highly recommended!

Bruce Caldwell

Retired High School Band Director,

Former Executive Manager WMEA, WMEA Hall of Fame,

Lesley's Dad

In this book, "I LOVE MY JOB BUT IT'S KILLING ME", the author Lesley Moffat explains through her own personal experiences of balancing a family life with a Commanding Career that there is "Light at the end of the tunnel". This book will take you on a journey from day to day ups and downs in real life. It will hit home for many readers. Personally, knowing the author for twenty plus years, she is and always will be a true inspiration to me! Lesley's devotion to life and now in writing this powerful book, she will show others how to make a heathier positive change in their own lives.

Thank you, my friend!

Pam Olson

I LOVE MY JOB BUT IT'S KILLING ME

I LOVE MY JOB BUT IT'S KILLING ME

The **TEACHER'S GUIDE** to Conquering **CHRONIC STRESS** and **SICKNESS**

LESLEY MOFFAT

NEW YORK

LONDON • NASHVILLE • MELBOURNE • VANCOUVER

I Love My Job But It's Killing Me
The Teacher's Guide to Conquering Stress and Sickness

Published in New York, New York, by Morgan James Publishing in partnership with Difference Press. Morgan James is a trademark of Morgan James, LLC. www.MorganJamesPublishing.com

ISBN 9781642796216 paperback
ISBN 9781642796223 eBook
Library of Congress Control Number: 2019943586

Interior Design by:
Christopher Kirk
www.GFSstudio.com

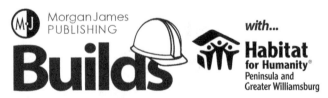

Morgan James is a proud partner of Habitat for Humanity Peninsula and Greater Williamsburg. Partners in building since 2006.

Get involved today! Visit
MorganJamesPublishing.com/giving-back

Foreword

Finding balance between one's personal and professional lives can be a difficult process for anyone, and when health issues rise to the level of undermining the work that needs to be done, the difficulty is exacerbated. In this book, Lesley Moffat recounts her personal journey as a high school band director, wife, and mother – a journey filled with many successes and reasons to celebrate, but also one marked by physical and mental health concerns, constant fatigue, multiple frustrations, and extreme stress.

When her best friend, Laurie, was diagnosed and subsequently succumbed to cancer, Lesley knew she had to find a way to balance the various aspects of her busy life and get her own health under control if she was going to be able to continue her career, be present for her family, and most important, live her life instead of just getting through it. Teachers tend to take care of others, often at the expense of their own well-being, and this certainly was the case for Lesley. She found herself sick of being sick all the time, worn down by visiting a plethora of health care professionals, and unable to understand the toll on her body as a result of the pharmaceuticals she was using to attempt to keep herself going.

While her approach is from the perspective of functioning as a female in the male-dominated world of band directing, the tools and strategies presented in this book should help anyone discover the joy gained from managing health and happiness in a way that provides renewed energy, better health, and sustainability in one's life work. She describes her own journey of self-awareness with abundant use of metaphors to help the reader understand concepts and relate them to their own careers and lives. She uses hands-on tools to show how through the use of mindfulness, music, movement, and meals, it is possible to create new and sustainable habits, live fully in the present, take care of oneself while being present for others, and create a new balance among the various aspects of life.

Lesley shares with readers the strategies and techniques that have worked for her in regaining her health and finding new pathways toward happiness and balance in her life. She encourages the reader to reach out for help, make these issues a priority, and create new habits that ensure a positive environment. While this kind of change does not come easily, it is inspiring to read her story and to examine how to apply her ideas to one's own life. For those who find themselves tired, stressed, unhealthy, and in need of balancing the various aspects of life, the tools are available and with discipline and commitment, it is possible to change your priorities and enjoy a more balanced and happy life. Lesley

Moffat skillfully shows how to make meaningful change and she is the living example of how her ideas can work.

–Nancy Ditmer
Professor of Music and Director of Bands,
The College of Wooster, Wooster, OH
Past President, Ohio Music Education Association
& National Association for Music Education (NAfME)

Dr. Laurie Cappello
May 20, 1957 – November 30, 2018
Friend, colleague, mentor, and teacher extraordinaire.
Hey you! Your legacy lives on....

Table of Contents

Introduction

*"Forgive yourself for not knowing
what you didn't know before you learned it."*
– Maya Angelou

The idea for this book came about because my dear friend Laurie and I spent time together as colleagues and friends for nearly two decades, sharing our joys and struggles as teachers, moms, and busy women. As women in the male-dominated field of high school band and choir directing, a friendship quickly developed between us as we leaned on each other for advice, encouragement, and support. Both of us were dealing with chronic health issues that impacted our abilities to do our jobs, not to mention our quality of life as we were overstressed, overscheduled, and over-exhausted.

We were both teaching music in large high schools with active and visible music programs that brought us incredible joy. Our days began long before the sun even thought about rising, our first classes starting at 6:30 every morning. We'd teach hundreds of kids throughout the course of each school day, followed by afternoons and evenings full of additional rehearsals, meetings, and performances. The constant go-go-go and do-more mentality began to take its toll on both of us, but we didn't know what to do.

We both dealt with joint pain and weight issues, had difficulty sleeping, and were often quite scatterbrained. We'd catch colds and other communicable diseases from our students because our own immune systems were being compromised the more worn-down we became. But in spite of the red flags our bodies were waving, we forged ahead.

And then came the phone call where Laurie told me she had Stage IV ovarian cancer. I remember pulling my car off the road and listening in shock with tears rolling down my cheeks as she said that the news was not good, but she was determined to fight it. And fight like heck she did – for over six years. I watched as she bravely faced each obstacle that came with that horrific disease, in awe of her strength and courage, but sad that she had to go through it.

She was so candid about what she was facing. As I was going through my own health challenges, we'd spend hours talking about how we got to such unhealthy places, and our conversations always came back to feeling like the stress of our jobs (much of which we admittedly brought on ourselves as we worked hard to build up our music programs) was ultimately putting a very real strain on our physical and mental well-being.

The phrase we both would say over and over was "I love my job, but it's killing me." That's how the title of this book came to be. It had become our mantra, and she begged me to find a way to take care of myself so I wouldn't end up in her shoes. In spite of her health crisis, it was Laurie who would check in with me to see how my hip replacement surgery went or how I'd recovered from my latest bout of pneumonia. And then she'd lovingly lecture me about slowing down and taking care of myself.

Laurie's life's work was to be a teacher. First and foremost, she taught kids. Through music, she taught them all kinds of life lessons about music, of course, but also about teamwork, setting goals, being responsible, looking out for each other, and a million other life skills. She helped them develop into compassionate and well-rounded individuals who could contribute to society.

Through this book, Laurie's legacy continues. I've taken the lessons I learned from her from the hundreds of hours we spent together during her chemo treatments, drives to her doctor appointments, and sitting in her family room, where we'd come to realize that in order for us to effectively do our jobs as teachers, we had to learn to take care of ourselves or we wouldn't have anything to give to our students. This book is a compilation of the lessons we learned together and information I've gathered from doctors and other health professionals as well as research I've done, reading everything I could get my hands on to find solutions to the health issues that had been plaguing me for decades.

Laurie encouraged me to write this book and share what we learned through our struggles and victories. She was my biggest cheerleader when I undertook this project, always checking in to make sure I was working on it. It's in her memory and honor that I offer this book in hopes it gives you the tools you need to reclaim your health so you can live the life you were meant to live.

As I write this introduction, I'm just hours away from uploading the entire manuscript. You see, the first draft of everything except the Introduction was finished three days ago, on the morning Laurie passed away, but I had not been able to write the intro at that point. The grief of her death is still very raw, but it's precisely because of the dire consequences we face when our health becomes so fragile that this message must be shared. Laurie wouldn't give up if she had an important lesson to share, so I must live up to her example and write it forward.

Laurie was and always will be a teacher. Her lessons are woven throughout this book. Her tenacity inspired me to take what we learned through our individual journeys and the lessons we've learned from almost twenty years of friendship and six decades of teaching between us and shout it from the mountaintops. If our message can be heard and used by even one person, then it will have mattered.

This book is a love letter to the women out there who are called to serve as teachers but who need a little extra help in caring for themselves so they have the energy and ability to take care of those they're privileged to teach. Teaching is an incredibly rewarding calling, but it's exhausting. May the tools you find in this book help you manage your health and happiness so you can get back to class and feel good again. After all, there are a lot of people depending on you – most of all, you. Let this book help you discover the joy of renewed energy, health, and sustainability in your life's work.

Chapter 1:

Where Am I?

*"You cannot escape a prison
if you do not know you're in one."*
– Vernon Howard

2:19 a.m. The glow of the blue light from the clock lets you know that there isn't much time left to get enough sleep to get you through your day ahead, but it's too early to get up and start. So you lie there, staring at the clock, with your to-do list popping up in your head like sticky notes whirling around your brain as if an industrial-strength fan is blowing them at full speed: Grocery shopping. Field trip paperwork to sign. House needs cleaning. Laundry's piled up. The car needs an oil change. Tuition for one of the kids is due next month. There are deadlines at work piling up faster than you can keep up. Doctor's appointments need to be made. So much yard work. That "one person" at work who gets under your skin. The list goes on and on and before you know it, your alarm's going off like a Mack truck heading straight at you. The constant chatter in your head robs you of peace of mind, sleep, and your ability to do your job. And now it's time to get up and start the routine that's been slowly making you sicker and sicker with each added responsibility and expectation until you're overwhelmed and under the weather. You really can't keep this up much longer, but what other option do you have?

The mornings start way too early. No matter what time you have to get up, you never feel rested and ready to go. Instead, the recent years have gradually become filled with more nights of restlessness rather than sleep, making it hard to get through your daily routines because your energy is zapped. The exhaustion is real – and it's mental and physical exhaustion. Your body is tired and hurting, which makes you avoid moving around too much because it's painful, and that doesn't allow you to do what you want and need to do, so your energy continues to wane as your anxiety about falling behind heightens. In the meantime, your capacity for decision-making and taking care of everyone else's needs has taken its toll on your mental health. You can feel yourself burning out in the things that used to bring you joy. You can barely drag yourself through your day, but the minute your head hits the pillow, *bam*, your eyes pop open, your brain revs up, and it doesn't look like you're getting to sleep any time soon.

Years or perhaps decades of this kind of living have made you sick and tired all the time, to the point that it interferes with your ability to do your job. It's probably hard to pinpoint the exact moment when you went from being in a place where you could balance the demands of your career and family life to being so overwhelmed that before you knew it, you were chronically ill with a myriad of symptoms. The things that contributed to getting you where you are probably came from every aspect of your life, and the impact of one "little" thing became much bigger than you realized it could be. Now you're wondering how to stop this craziness. It might feel like you're in the middle of a snow globe. Just like the scene inside a snow globe, your goals aren't visible through all the mental and physical clutter that gets in your way. It feels impossible to know where to start or what to do to get control over your life again, so you just keep plugging away, but every day gets harder and harder and you know your current pace of life isn't really sustainable.

It may have started with physical pain. Maybe the pain was becoming too much to bear, so the monthly prescriptions of opioid pain meds became a necessity in order to function at work or at home. The tradeoff to using pain meds was the havoc it wreaked on the rest of your body, and so began the downward spiral of prescription after prescription to take care of all of the ailments that began to pop up. Medicine to help you go to sleep, then another prescription to help you *stay* asleep, followed by more pills in the morning for your ADHD – an amphetamine and "upper" to help you stay awake – then the anti-inflammatories, anti-depressants, and anti-anxiety meds to help with a myriad of other symptoms. The list goes on and on, as do the conditions for which they are being prescribed. And now you may be realizing that many of the medications you are taking are to counteract the side effects of other prescriptions you are on. Is more of the same really an option anymore?

When is enough, enough? Did everything seem to sneak up on you and before you knew it you had a ton of responsibilities that left little time to take care of your own needs and passions? Is all this giving to others taking a toll on your health? When do you get to take the advice of the FAA and "put on your own oxygen mask" before putting on anyone else's, or are you constantly taking care of everyone else's needs to the point where you have nothing left for yourself?

And you are sick and tired of being sick and tired, but you're too tired to do anything about it because there's another "more important" job that has to be done first. And then another. And another. It never stops. But your body is wearing out. You can't keep up at this pace. You're missing more and more work for health issues that never quite seem to go away. And even when you are at work, your mind isn't fully present. There are other pressing needs that draw your attention and energy, sucking the life out of you.

And the exhaustion. Can we talk about the exhaustion? There's never a time of day or night when it feels like you have the kind of energy you need to do the task at hand, whether that's teaching an engaging lesson to a class full of teenagers or settling down and going to sleep, so you feel like you're in a fog all the time. And an exhausted body doesn't fight off germs, so you're always getting hit with the latest colds, infections, and other communicable diseases, and it just keeps getting worse.

You invested a lot of energy, time, money, and passion into a career that you truly love, but now you're finding it's becoming too difficult to continue at the rate you've been going. And maybe your energies are being sucked into activities that don't serve you well. Who knew raising a family and working in such a demanding and intense job could be so taxing? Does it seem improbable if not impossible that you can ever regain the vitality and health you used to have so you can finish out your career with a bang instead of a fizzle? You've got a lot riding on this – all you've done to establish yourself in your chosen field has been your life's work, so just walking away isn't an option, but neither is continuing to miss work for weeks at a time or being so sick and miserable that you aren't able to be fully engaged in anything you are doing. That's not healthy for anyone, and it's certainly not sustainable.

There is a better way, and you can experience it, but only if you know what steps to take. That's where this book comes in. It is your guide to assessing what steps you need to take in order to get back to that place where you feel in control and have the energy to do what you need to do – and maybe even what you *want* to do, too! There is hope, and by picking up this book and reading this far, you've just taken the first step in finding the path for getting healthy enough to go back to work and not get sick all the time.

Chapter 2:

How Did I Get Here?

*"Sometimes what you're most afraid of doing
is the very thing that will set you free."*
– Robert Tew

Think about the last time you felt good about being you. When you didn't feel like you had to do something to make someone else happy, but that you could make a decision that made you feel good. When did you have fun doing something you did because you wanted to? I'm not talking about having fun volunteering for a favorite charity or a good time working on a project for your job, I'm talking about something that fed your soul. Something that made you lose track of time because you were so in the moment. Is it hard to think of even one example, at least one from any time in the recent past?

Do you feel like you have to put everyone else's needs above your own? Have you found your health to be suffering yet no matter how many times you go to the doctor and get new medication, you don't seem to get any better? Are you finding it hard to admit that a million little things snuck up on you and now you're to the point where you can't keep up? Or maybe you don't want to keep up anymore because it's taking such a toll on your health, both physically and mentally. When you take stock of the things you've tried to solve your health problems in the past, do you see a pattern of sinking your money, time, and energy into Band-Aid type temporary fixes or long-term sustainable changes that helped you get healthy? Does it feel like a never-ending battle of trying to mask symptoms without any real relief? Have you had doctors tell you that the late-night panic attacks, weight gain, headaches, exhaustion, insomnia, pain, and other symptoms are "just stress"?

Well, this stuff's for real – and it's killing you. I know this because it was killing me and I am seeing what it's doing to my colleagues, friends, and students. I watched cancer rob my best friend of growing old with her husband and being around her first grandchild because the stress of her job manifested itself in her body as a vicious illness. The high school students I teach are experiencing more and more mental health crises, and their parents are beyond stressed as they work multiple jobs, try to raise their families, and keep up with all the demands on their time.

And look at what it's doing to you. You've picked up this book because you realize you have to do something drastically different or you are going to end up having to say goodbye to finishing out your career or give up on fulfilling those dreams you put on hold for so many years because you were taking care of everyone else. When is it going to be your turn to do what you want to do? How about *now*? Like, today – this very minute? You've already had the good sense to search for a resource to help you change the path you're on, so why not take a few more steps with me and be curious about what kind of journey is possible for you?

Our weight does not define us. That said, our weight is a direct reflection of what was going on in our minds and bodies. As I look back, the times when I struggled the most were times when I was at my heaviest. My body was responding to the food I ate and the stressful conditions to

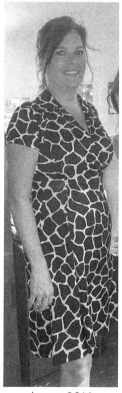
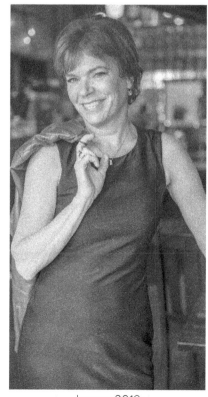

August 2016   January 2019

which I subjected it. It was uncomfortable, awkward, and unhealthy. My skin was dry and my hair felt like straw. I had acne. My joints hurt because it was hard to carry the extra weight. It didn't feel good to have my clothes dig into my skin or my thighs rubbing together. And when I was heavier, I was always sick. Sometimes it was a cold or other virus, but often times it was much worse. Looking back, I realize there was a lot of toxic stuff in my body and it was literally weighing me down.

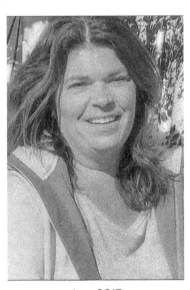
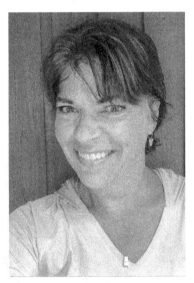

June 2017   June 2018

This is me at various points in my life. In 2017, I was a hot mess. At 5'7" and 200 pounds, I had arthritis, ADHD, horrible brain fog, chronic exhaustion, migraines, and replacement body parts in my hip, back, and neck. I was on a toxic cocktail of pharmaceuticals to "keep me healthy," but it only made me sicker in the long run. Fast-forward to today – I'm still 5'7," but at 135 pounds, I'm off all the pharmaceuticals, I have more energy than I had in my thirties, and I feel like I've gotten a new lease on life. The chronic health conditions I'd dealt with for decades are *gone*!

The visible changes in me are nothing compared to the changes that took place inside my mind and body. Through research, trial and error, and lots of hard work, I have transformed from being unhealthy and exhausted to having energy and clarity that sustains me in a new way. I have a renewed zest for life and want to share this plan with everyone who is ready to own their future.

This book is about discovering *what you need* and *how to get what you need*. In this book, we will look at what it is that is making you feel the need to seek change. We'll discover how your lifestyle choices impact your life. I'll teach you how to transform from being sick and tired to not only being healthy enough to return to work without getting sick again, but to reignite that passion and drive that somehow went missing when you were busy living life.

You'll feel an amazing transformation take place as your symptoms begin to subside, weight falls off effortlessly (I am serious about this part), and your energy returns with a vengeance. I am living proof of these statements, and I want to show you how you can reclaim your quality of life.

I've created this practical guide in the same way I've designed lessons for my high school band students for the past thirty-one years, with straightforward assessments of your current situation, the understanding of your specific goals, and creation of a plan that will work for transforming *you* into the healthy and happy woman you deserve to be. We will do this step-by-step, and by creating a plan that works for *you*, it'll be sustainable because it'll be what *you* need.

As Dr. Seuss would say, "Congratulations, today is *your* day. You're off to great places. You're off and away!" If you've gotten this far in the book, then you know that it's *your* turn – right now. You don't have to ask yourself if you're ready to make a change because you've already started. Just now. Today. This very minute. You already took the first step. The hardest step. You are no longer going to be a victim of your circumstances. You've taken action and I'm here to be by your side every step of the way.

Remember what it was like when you were at the height of your career and family life? When things might have been busy, but at least they were manageable? Perhaps even joyful? It is going to feel fantastic when you get back to that place where you are in your flow, where your body and mind feel fresh and alert, and where you can feel good about being you. When you feel that joy in living a healthy life again, you'll find a renewed zest for everything you do, and it'll feel really frickin' amazing!

I've spent over three decades teaching high school band. It is my job to convince up to seventy-five teenagers at a time who have noisemakers in their hands to work with one another toward a common goal (perhaps a concert at Carnegie Hall) where they will go demonstrate what they have learned in a concert in front of thousands of people from all over the world. Kids ranging in age from fourteen to eighteen who are just regular students in a public high school (this is not a magnet school for music) have performed three times so far at Carnegie Hall under my leadership, with additional performances all over the US, Canada, and on Royal Caribbean cruise ships, as well as Disneyland and other theme parks.

In order for my students to be successful in efforts of this magnitude, I must be able to assess each of their individual strengths, weaknesses, and goals. I need to evaluate what kind of key information is needed to get the student to the next level, and if I need to design a special lesson or rewrite a part so it's accessible to a student, then I do it. This book works the same way. Instead of a one-size-fits-all solution, it has been designed to help you identify *your* individual needs and goals and the best way for *you* to reach them.

I'll be here to help you discover how to break through the barriers that have kept you from completely healing no matter what you've tried. I've got ideas and advice for making real changes that stick. I've got the experience of working with thousands of people and helping them reach their potential and beyond. And I want to help you because I've been exactly where you are, and it sucks. So let's go. If you're ready to change your life and not look back, take a deep breath, exhale, and turn the page. It's about to get real!

Chapter 3:

My Journey

"When you're in a dark place,
you tend to think you've been buried –
perhaps you've been planted ... bloom!"
– Christine Caine

I went to see my family doctor in February of 2017. My list of complaints was long. I hardly knew where to begin. Working fifty plus hours per week at the career of my dreams while raising a family was taking its toll on me. My forties were supposed to be rewarding and fulfilling, I had worked my backside off for decades to get where I was, but it seemed all I'd experienced for the previous twenty-nine years had been exhaustion and one health crisis after another. And now I was convinced I had early-onset dementia. I couldn't focus or remember anything, and being on the highest dose allowable of medication for ADHD wasn't helping me.

Then there was the weight gain. The weight had slowly crept up on me, and by the time I hit my darkest point, I was 200 pounds, miserable, unhealthy, in pain, and physically and mentally exhausted. I stopped going to work. My gut was a mess and it made everything else feel awful. For two months, I remained a recluse in my home, barely leaving my back deck. I couldn't function. Everything hurt. I couldn't stand eating because I was nauseous all the time and when I did eat, I ended up vomiting a lot.

"It's probably stress," all the doctors keep saying, making me feel like it was something I should be able to manage on my own. It never felt like anyone could understand what I was experiencing. But the physical and mental fatigue were real. The pneumonia, back surgery, neck surgery, gallbladder removal, hysterectomy, hip replacement, bunion removal, restless leg syndrome, migraines, other illnesses, and inability to focus were real. The pain from arthritis and other things never seemed to get better, so turning to medication for relief in order to function became part of my daily routine.

Then there was the ADHD. How could I possibly focus on anything when I was constantly being bombarded by the stimulation of band instruments, drums, and the sheer number of people for whom I was responsible every single hour of every single day? With hundreds of teenagers in my classes hour after hour, day after day, and my own husband, children, extended family, and friends to tend to, it was no wonder I was crashing and burning.

Over the course of my career I've experienced much joy. I teach in a homey suburb where my husband and I raised our kids. For twelve consecutive years, I had one of my girls in one or more of my classes every day. My parents live close by and helped out all the time. The community and school are ideal places to live and work. I live in the neighborhood I serve, giving me the opportunity to get to know my students and their families not only as a teacher, but also through church and other community activities. My students and their families are also friends of our family. The support for our music program is phenomenal, and it's because of the amazing students and parents who are a part of the music family. But in spite of all the support, I was still struggling.

When I went to the doctor on that day in 2017, life was quite good for the most part, but there was something missing. I was under more and more pressure to have the band do more – why can't they go to more sporting events or an additional field trip or do another community service activity – and it was wearing me down. My responsibilities took their toll on my health. Taking care of myself hadn't been on my radar for years, and my body, mind, and spirit were deteriorating.

Like you, my days are packed. My career began simply enough, and then came my own kids. And then more demands. By the age of thirty-two, I'd just had my third child (in September, right after school started, which meant monitoring a substitute teacher while also being the mom to two young children and a new baby during my short maternity leave). Returning to school, I was back to a grueling schedule once again. With the help of my husband, we had to get the three girls up and get ready for the day, getting everyone out the door by 5:45 every morning. Before leaving the house, I had to get everyone ready, nurse the baby, pump more milk for her to have during the day, pack the pump so I could pump during my planning period, pack all the things the kids needed for school and daycare, and get my things together for school. I would already be worn out before I'd stepped out the door or a single student had walked into my classroom.

This profession is hard. Until my generation, women weren't high school band directors, so there were no role models for me to look up to when I struggled with finding a balance between raising a family and having this career path. I had to learn things the hard way and make up my own solutions when there weren't resources for me to use.

My peer group is primarily men. How could my male band directing colleagues relate to my struggles? They may have kids, but they didn't have to spend nine months making those babies while teaching (an exhausting combination that cost me a miscarriage during a band trip), and then pump breast milk during their planning periods to feed each of those babies for the first six months of their lives. And how many of them had to ask a spouse to make a ninety-minute drive with their newborn baby in the car behind the school buses where the band had to play for basketball playoffs so they could nurse the baby in the bathroom when they weren't directing the band? The additional responsibilities I had simply because I'd chosen to be a mom in addition to being a band teacher made it harder for me to be part of the "good old boys club" that seemed to make up the bulk of the high school band directors, and that isolation only contributed to my declining health.

I loved so many things about being a high school band director. My dad had been my high school band director and since I grew up around the band kids and all the activities they did, there was never any doubt about following in my dad's footsteps of being a high school band director in the community where my own kids attended school. His bands were the talk of the town and were always performing at everything from concerts and festivals to high school football games and multiple Presidential Inaugurations. The bands were visible in the school and community and they played everywhere.

And my mom was perfect. Even though she was a full-time teacher who was also raising my brother and sister and me, she made it look easy. She sewed clothes for the family. There was a hot meal on the table every night and everyone sat down at the table for dinner together. The laundry never piled up. She always had plenty of energy to help with homework, volunteer with the PTA, and pretty much be like Mary Poppins. How the heck could I live up to those kinds of standards? I felt like I had to be the best mom *and* the best high school band director. Period. I had to be as good as each of them, and that was going to prove to be a futile task. But I had chosen this path, so I certainly wasn't about to admit it was hard. It was very hard. It was killing me.

As my health gradually began deteriorating, I became more and more reliant on medications just to get from day to day. The cocktail of drugs, ironically paid for by my employer in the job that was driving the declining health issues, included meds for ADHD, sleeping pills to help me fall asleep, anti-psychotic drugs to help me stay asleep when my to-do lists kept my brain alert all night, meds to keep my restless leg syndrome under control so my legs wouldn't kick all night, anti-inflammatories for arthritis, opioids for severe pain after surgery and chronic pain, and much more had come about as a result of the Band-Aid approach to healthcare. Every trip to the doctor with a complaint resulted in a new prescription to mask the latest symptom. And the side effects of each of these drugs were turning out to be worse than the original symptoms, but getting to the root cause was a luxury I didn't have because that would take time and I didn't have time. I had to power through because there were so many demands being placed on me. Time was not my own.

Even with the massive amounts of meds being used to help me sleep, sleep had still been elusive much of the time. Those late nights were made worse because of the nonstop narrative in my head. "Things would be so much better, *if only…*" and the lists would be long. *If only* I didn't have so many demands on my time and energy. *If only* I wasn't always getting sick. *If only* my peers, mostly males, respected me. *If only* that *one* parent or student would change. *If only* I had more time. *If only*…. And then the alarm would go off, jolting me into another jam-packed day of taking care of everyone else's needs … and another day of putting my own needs on the back burner.

There's a reason flight attendants instruct us to put on our own oxygen mask before assisting others. I always felt that was a terribly selfish thing to do. After all, I love my kids so much I would do anything to save them, including giving them an oxygen mask before taking care of myself. I approached my teaching and family life with that same mindset, believing I had to put everyone else's needs first and then take care of myself if, and only if, there was time (and resources.) That meant I was saying yes to other people's requests when I really should have been saying no, and then finding myself overextended and unappreciated for my efforts. And I always ended up saying no to myself when I really deserved to say yes. This cycle of pleasing other people was taking its toll.

That's why I went to see my doctor that day in 2017. Since I hadn't put on my own proverbial oxygen mask, I had run out of my own fuel and no longer had anything to give to others. In order for me to serve my students, I had to take care of myself so I would be able to be present and have something to give to them. When I realized I was being sent back for another cycle of running more tests and taking more drugs, I just couldn't face it again. The same old routine wasn't going to work this time any better than it had worked in the past. My best friend was dying of cancer and we had spent hours talking about stress and its effect on our health. I had to do something drastically different or I wouldn't be far behind her.

If I was going to continue in this profession without burning out or becoming so sick that I had to quit, then something had to change *now*. I was at the end of my rope. And so, I am guessing, are you.

After a long and often discouraging search for how I could regain my health and vitality and get back to the job I love, I have come to a place where I've found peace and health and happiness. I am back in my classroom every day with a renewed vigor and vitality, feeling in the flow, and my work feels effortless. But it wasn't a quick fix or easy road. It took a lot of patience, time, and trial and error to learn the strategies I needed to employ in my life if I was going to experience meaningful and sustainable change. It required me to dig deep and become aware of the impact my actions have had on my body and mind and then learn how to address them.

There have been tears of frustration, joy, and everything in between. It has been hard, but it has been so worth it. I have come to understand what it takes to fix the body and mind so they can sustain me through the work I need and want to do. I am off of *all* of the pharmaceuticals I'd been taking for decades, and I feel free. I am driven to share my passion with students in my classroom as their music teacher and with women like you who, after decades of serving other people, need a little guidance in what steps to take to regain your own health so you can get back to your purpose-driven life and fulfill your goals.

This book will help you do just that. With my help, you'll learn to do the things that will bring you the health and peace of mind you crave and deserve. You'll find practical and doable tips that don't cost anything to implement but that have immediate and permanent positive benefits. You'll learn how to cope with setbacks and what they teach you about moving forward. And you'll be empowered to live the life you dreamed you'd be living, without chronic health issues getting in the way.

So let's get started, because the journey to a new you begins right now!

Chapter 4:

Let's Get Started!

"One day you'll wake up and realize this isn't what you want to feel like anymore and you'll be done!"
– Bri Lamper

Once you *know* better, you can *do* better. I created the mPower Method as a program to help women who are struggling with their health due to the demands of their careers and raising a family. It came about as the result of what I learned and discovered about how to overcome the physical and emotional challenges that are inherent with being a mom and a high school band director. I didn't have many women as role models in this kind of job who were raising a family of their own, so it often felt like I was alone in my struggles. Once I realized how many other teachers are in the same boat, I knew I had to share what I'd learned like I wish someone could have done for me all those years ago. I took inventory of what I'd done to reclaim my health and did what any teacher would do: created a way to teach it to others.

The mPower Method has four key components; meals, movement, music, and mindfulness. You will be taking an assessment (the Mojo Meter) to identify areas in which you need to make changes. Then we will look at various tools and techniques you can employ to make those changes happen. Based on your responses, you'll find out why and how the meals you eat, movement you make, music you listen to or perform, and mindfulness you incorporate in your daily life are the foundation of a healthy and sustainable future. You'll be able to develop a plan that works with your particular situation and needs, and you will discover concrete steps you can take to achieve your goals. You'll find tips you can use in your classroom to manage many of the things that add stress to your already overwhelming responsibilities.

My SNaP Strategies (Start Now and Progress) give you examples of ways to develop new skills by changing habits one step at a time. And there are plenty of tips for replacing habits that no longer serve you with the ones that support you in the goals you are setting for yourself. You can use this list as a starting point and add whatever ideas fit your life.

This book is a tool for you to use to personalize your own plan. By doing the homework and diving into the Action Plans at the end of the chapters, you'll be on your way to creating the change you crave. There's no time like the present to take that first step, so let's go.

Here's the Mojo Meter. Go ahead and take the assessment. Don't fuss a lot about your answers. Go with your first instinct and move on. Your gut will know the answer that really applies, but if you think it through too much, you'll convince yourself to answer the way you think you should and then the results won't help you make the changes you crave.

Moffat's Mojo Meter:

1. I have a lot of aches and pains.   T   F

2. I often feel tired after eating.   T   F

3. My memory doesn't seem to be as sharp as it used to be.   T   F

4. Other people have mentioned that I seem down, upset, or not myself.   T   F

5. I experience a lot of brain fog.   T   F

6. I don't have enough energy to get me through my days without it being a struggle.   T   F

7. I experience digestive issues several times a week.   T   F

8. I feel tired a lot of the time.   T   F

9. I get a lot of illnesses, like colds, sinus infections, and other common and contagious ailments.   T   F

10. I don't have any energy in reserve.   T   F

11. My weight is higher than what feels good.   T   F

12. I experience frequent bloating.   T   F

13. Sometimes I feel like all I want to do is cry and escape the exhaustion.   T   F

14. I am at a weight that doesn't feel good.   T   F

15. I don't have a regular (4+ times per week) exercise routine.   T   F

16. My desk / workspace feels cluttered.   T   F

17. My house feels cluttered.   T   F

18. My closets are disorganized.   T   F

19. Even though I like my job, I often dread going to work.   T   F

20. My car is messy.   T   F

21. I feel like there's never enough time to get things done.   T   F

22. My mind could be described as a snow globe that's been shaken up.   T   F

23. Sometimes just getting through the day is a huge chore.   T   F

24. I have trouble falling asleep several times a week.   T   F

25. I have trouble staying asleep.   T   F

26. I feel overwhelmed more and more often.   T   F

27. It's getting harder and harder to keep up at the pace I'm living.   T   F

28. I feel like no one understands all the things I'm juggling.   T   F

29. I love my family but their needs are draining my energy.   T   F

30. I love my job, but it's taking a toll on my health and life.   T   F

31. I feel like everything is spinning out of control, and I kind of don't even care anymore.   T   F

32. There are a few people who drive me crazy.   T   F

33. Social media often gets me upset.   T   F

34. My newsfeed is full of bad and discouraging news.   T   F

35. I feel angry and frustrated a lot.   T   F

36. I don't have energy to do the things I love.   T   F

37. My sex drive is pretty much blah.   T   F

38. I have given up doing a lot of the things that used to make me happy.   T   F

39. I often feel like I'm surviving instead of thriving.   T   F

40. I don't have at least one just-for-me activity (hobby or something I do at least once a week for my own personal enjoyment).   T   F

Before we go any further, I need you to think about how you are going to approach this lifestyle shift. If you are in a hurry to get another short-term fix, then you aren't ready to continue, but if you are looking for a sustainable way to literally turn back the clock and reclaim your life so you can fully participate in all the joys it has to offer, then buckle up, because your mind is about to be blown!

If you're ready to proceed, then look at the Mojo Meter and tally your score.

How many statements were true for you? _____

How many were false? __

If you found ten or fewer of these statements to be true for you, then congratulations, you are probably managing pretty well. You can read the suggestions in this book that address the areas in which you are looking for improvement and likely meet with success, and as your situation changes, you can always refer to chapters that are relevant for whatever you are facing to enlist new strategies if needed.

If you answered true to eleven or more of these statements, then I know why you are here. I understand the struggle, and I know how hard it is to know where to start. By looking at the areas where you are facing the toughest challenges, you can find steps to take to make changes *now*. It's time to reclaim your health and energy, so get ready to amaze yourself.

We are going to explore various techniques for making positive changes in the areas where you are struggling the most. Much like the process of learning to play an instrument, changing habits and behaviors takes daily practice over a period of time. It requires a commitment to doing something that might feel awkward or unusual at first, but if you stick with the plan, you will amaze yourself with the results. You will see *impossible* transform to *I'm possible.*

The only way for you to grow is to confront whatever is holding you back and then replace that behavior or habit with a better option. You've just identified the consequences of all the stress, exhaustion, and illness in your life through your answers in your Mojo Meter. For every statement you answered as true, you identified the very building blocks for the challenges you're facing. You can probably already see some areas where you are going to want to make changes as soon as possible.

Making a big life change is scary – but what's even scarier is *not* making a change when the alternative to change is continued illness or worse. You are going to learn how to be the leader of your life, putting your needs in the proper priority order. In fact, you just might find yourself with renewed vigor along with a healthier you. What's not to love about all that?

You love your job (or at least most aspects of your job), so that may make it hard to admit that it is causing you stress. I couldn't acknowledge the stress for most of my life because doing so would have made me appear or feel weak, and that wasn't an option. But whether or not I was willing to admit there was a lot of stress involved in my job, *it was definitely there.*

As brain research tells us, stress wreaks havoc on our minds and bodies. The constant stimulation from electronic devices, social media, traffic, and everything else we encounter in our world every day is literally making us sick.

Add to that a classroom full of students with instruments in their hands and you've got an even more over-stimulating environment from which you rarely get a break.

Even if we don't feel stressed, our bodies are victims of all this bombardment to our senses. Massive amounts of cortisol are being released into our bloodstreams round the clock, but that hormone is really intended to save our lives in a fight-or-flight situation. The result of this kind of constant exposure to cortisol manifests itself in the forms of feeling like you are always in a mental fog, having difficulty falling or staying asleep, being sick a lot, having constant aches and pains, lacking energy, feeling exhausted and emotional, and wondering how much longer you can hold it together.

The only way to get out of the constant spiral of ill-nesses, catching every bug that comes through your class-room, doctor visits, temporary relief, then repeating that cycle over and over again is to change something. Whatever you're doing now isn't working, so you must do something different if you're going to get different results.

No one ever trips over a mountain. It's the smaller rocks and stones along the way that cause them to fall. Life's a lot like that – we work so hard at making those big moments happen that in the process we trip and fall while we are trying to get to our proverbial mountains. Your answers to the Mojo Meter will help you identify the rocks that are tripping you up and determine which ones need to be addressed, stepped over, or be completely released from your path.

I spend a lot of time outside on my deck. I didn't used to do that. I was too busy… or so I thought. As I marvel at nature, I have learned some pretty important lessons, perhaps the most important being that no matter what I do with my plants, if I put them in soil that isn't full of the nutrients they need, they don't stand a chance of surviving very long. I know this because I have *plenty* of experience with what happens to lovely flowers that are transplanted into cheap dirt. They die. No amount of water or fancy fertilizer can revive a plant that is suffocating in dirt. And neither can people. Neither can you.

Just like plants grow in soil through which they receive their nourishment, so, too, do we. We are nourished by the habits that create an environment in which we either thrive or we don't. Our output is directly related to our input. Garbage in equals garbage out. If flowers are planted in dirt that doesn't have what they need, they die. If you and I are allowing garbage of any kind into our lives, whether through what we eat, watch, read, or discuss, then all we can do is regurgitate it and make garbage to send out. It appears in the form of illnesses, negative thoughts, bad feelings, missed days of work, depression, anxiety, and more.

What we put in ourselves isn't limited to food and drinks. It includes how we stimulate our minds. Are you spending your time doing things that are positive, healthy, and in your best interest or are you getting sucked into social media battles, complaining about your situation, or anticipating more bad luck? Like it or not, every action, thought, and bit of nourishment you take in has some kind of impact on you. Period. So now it's time to identify how the choices you make impact you and then decide if you want to continue with those feelings or change them. It's that simple. Really.

I'm a firm believer in the Law of Attraction. I was a skeptic for quite a while, especially when I was at my worst.

After all, I had a long list of what was going wrong with my body and how stressed I was at work and dozens of other reasons why the Law of Attraction didn't work. I wanted to feel good, but I continued to feel crappy, so that law didn't apply to me. Or so I thought.

The principle of the Law of Attraction is simple: Like attracts like. Much like a mirror, what we see and hear and notice around us is a reflection of how we feel on the inside. I really understood this universal law when reflecting on one of my classes last year. It is an advanced percussion ensemble with twenty of the most musically talented kids around. Most of my classes have sixty to seventy-five students in them, so this one group of twenty should have been a breeze to manage. After all, I was pretty darn good at classroom management with the large ensembles, so I was befuddled as to why this particular class was driving me nuts. It used to be my favorite class of the day. The older students were amazing leaders who had mentored the younger kids and the quality of their music improved year after year, but the past year the environment had turned toxic and I couldn't figure out why. I tried positive reinforcement, natural consequences, assigning them to various small groups, and every other teacher-trick I knew, yet no matter how well they could each play their individual parts, they just couldn't gel as a unit.

We spent a lot of time talking about why we couldn't get in our groove, and it finally dawned on me. I had to take a look at what I was seeing and analyze it. Unintentionally, I had created a culture that had become toxic. My classroom was a reflection of what I was doing as the teacher, so I had to look in the mirror and see why the kids were acting the way they were. The Law of Attraction was at work right under my nose – the very anxieties with which I was dealing (feeling overwhelmed and out of control) were manifesting themselves in my students' behaviors as I created an environment where everyone was trying to be in charge and take control.

I had spent a lot of time working at cultivating a culture of student leadership. I took great pride in the fact that students took ownership of what we did, so I naturally encouraged that kind of behavior. I did such a good job of this that suddenly I had an entire class full of people trying to be leaders. I'd completely turned the culture upside down and in that class there was no one who was willing to follow other leaders. In my attempt to initially cultivate a culture of leadership, I had gone overboard and we ended up with twenty "leaders." I realized their behaviors were a reflection of what I had modeled and encouraged, and while my intent had been good, this class needed to learn different skill sets in order to accomplish their goal of being a cohesive unit both musically and interpersonally. I had to change what I taught them if they were going to have different results.

Once we identified that as our core issue, we knew where to begin. I let them know that while I really appreciated the leadership skills they were developing, we were going to shift gears and I was taking the lead. In order to build their teamwork skills, I incorporated activities that required them to work together and problem-solve in completely different ways than they had been doing. From the time we identified the core problem in February until the state music competition in April, our focus was as much on reestablishing our culture as it was on preparing the music. The result of reflecting on root cause and addressing the changes that needed to be made turned the group around 180 degrees, creating bonds that are stronger than any of us could have anticipated and resulting in them earning three perfect scores at the state music competition. By focusing on our core relationships and being mindful of the "rocks," we were able to shift our momentum *and* improve the learning and performing of music at the same time. It took hard work and daily practice of our teamwork skills, but by the time we changed our habits for a few weeks, new and better results were already evident, and once the kids felt the difference, they worked harder at building the new culture. The same thing will happen to you. As soon as you make small changes, you'll start to notice differences. One positive change will lead to another and the Law of Attraction will take you in a new direction! But first you need to take the time to figure out how you got where you are and why that isn't working. By identifying your goals and what is truly keeping you from reaching them, you can make a plan to fight for them, to successfully return to your more vibrant and healthy self.

You will be successful in transforming from the place you are in now back to your more vibrant and healthy self if you take the time to really look at how you got where you are and why it isn't working. By identifying your goals and what is truly keeping you from reaching them you are then able to make a plan for getting there.

In my work with clients, this is where the real transformation takes place. When we dig in and start with root-cause of what's really getting in their way, the other stuff falls into place quickly and permanently. In fact, within the first week of our one-on-one work together, my clients have sent me texts saying, "I want to thank you for helping people help themselves. You are such an inspiration to me." "I had the best day yesterday that I've had in months and months. Thank you!" and "When I went to church this morning, someone said I looked more peppy, like the me they used to know!" The reason they say this is because we start by working on getting them to feel better. You know how it is – when you feel better, you want to do better, and then you attract more good feelings and the Law of Attraction begins to shift your energy and how things play out in your life to align with things that make you feel good. It's addicting. You can experience this by following the mPower Method I created.

The next several chapters will take you through the process of reflecting and planning. Take the time to do the exercises and go to the links with the videos that supplement this book. Use all the resources available to really learn what makes you tick and how to keep it going. This shouldn't be a chore. It should be an opportunity to do what you should have done a long time ago – show yourself the same kind of love and compassion you've been showing everyone else for years and years. You deserve it.

Simply reading the information and suggestions will not suffice. There is no overnight solution – after all, you didn't get where you are overnight, so be patient with yourself as you begin this journey. If you had a friend or family member who was struggling like you are, you would encourage her to take care of herself, so take your own advice and stick with this. Surround yourself with people who will support you in the same way you support others. Find someone to help hold you accountable because it will be tough, but it's possible to experience change and *you* can do it.

Stick with it. Follow the recommendations as we explore your particular health issues and the solutions you can implement. There will be opportunities for you to assess where you are and where you want to be and then see how you can support those goals through your meal choices, the movement you incorporate into your daily routine, the music you listen to or play, and how mindfully approaching this process is the key to making it successful.

Some of the suggestions may seem silly or distracting at first, but hang in there because you will discover they are exercises in teaching your mind to be present in the moment, a practice of being mindful of what is happening and how it makes you feel. *It is this skill that will make choosing your meals, movement, and music much easier by helping you recognize and align those choices with what you feel and experience.*

At the end of each of the chapters that outline the mPower Method, you'll find an Action Plan (homework) to help you put what you are learning into action. These action plans are the way you track and see your progress. They also provide an opportunity for you to reflect on your progress and see patterns that support you in your endeavors and identify the things that are barriers to your success. Just find a way that works for you to keep these plans handy as a reference. *How* you do it isn't as important as the fact that you are doing it. This will become a powerful tool for tracking your progress.

Chapter 5:

The mPower Method –
Meals

"The secret of change is to focus all of your energy,
not on fighting the old, but on building the new."
– Socrates

A car can't go anywhere without fuel, no matter how fabulous and expensive the car is. The same is true for you. You must have your fuel, which is food, in order to function. There is a direct correlation between the type and quality of food you consume and every aspect of your health. Period. For fifty-one years, I firmly believed it was healthiest to stick to the traditional food pyramid, which was built on a diet of starches and carbs and low in fats, but look where that got me. I also fell for the rationale that my weight was a direct result of the number of calories I consumed. I had no clue that the *quality* of the calories played a bigger role in everything from my weight to my quality of life than the *number* of calories. Once I understood and embraced the truth that what I'd been doing for five decades wasn't working for me, my life changed.

My initial goal when I began the healing part of my journey was just to feel well enough to work without getting sick again. Feeling *great* wasn't even on my radar. I had hoped to be on a fraction of the medications I was on at the time, never dreaming that I would be weaned off *all* of the pharmaceuticals I'd been on for decades. And being 5'7" and 200 pounds when I was sickest, it never dawned on me that within months I would weigh 135 pounds and wear a size 4 – and that I would have abs and a toned body simply through the gentle practices of yoga and walking. If I had been told that my ADHD symptoms would be gone *and* my memory would be sharper than it had been in twenty years, I'd have laughed at the ridiculousness of that possibility.

I had *no* idea what was in store for me, but I'm certainly glad I hit rock-bottom so I could begin my journey out of the downward spiral into which I had fallen. It was through this experience that the four cornerstones of my mPower Method evolved, the result of my own assessment and discovery of what was causing me to feel so horrible and what was helping me feel and function better. Once I finally figured out what had been such a mystery to me for so many years, I knew I had to share it with others who were going through the same suffocating experience.

The first component of my mPower Method is *meals*. The meals you eat are the basis of everything from how you feel to how you function. What you put in your body literally *becomes* your body. Our cells are regenerating constantly. Think about it – if you are eating foods that have been treated with pesticides, are filled with artificial ingredients, and have antibiotics and other hormones added to them, then those things are all going into your body. Your body isn't meant to use these things in productive ways that help you grow, heal, think, and function, so many of the processes your body goes through become impeded and don't work like they should.

Years and even decades of eating stuff that didn't benefit my body took its toll in the form of excess weight, acne, dry skin, memory loss, brain fog, ADHD, pain, repeated infections, infertility, and dozens of other ailments. I had gotten to the point where I figured I was so far gone with such a long list of health problems that there was no turning things around, so I was about to settle for just "not getting any worse," but eventually I realized that option really sucked. Why should I succumb to being sick, tired, overweight, in pain, and feeling like crap when there might be a different possibility out there? After all, I was only 51 at the time. I wasn't ready to throw in the towel, so I figured it was now or never and I took a leap of faith and never looked back.

We have been taught in the past that we should be eating lots of fruits, veggies, and nonfat foods and avoiding fats. Our diets are inundated with sugars, grain, additives, preservatives, added hormones, and all kinds of other things our bodies weren't made to process, so our bodies respond with aches and pains or brain fog in hopes of getting our attention and letting us know what we are doing isn't working. When we ignore those symptoms, our bodies have to do something more drastic to get our attention so we will stop doing the things that are making us sick. I didn't get the message until my body was riddled with all kinds of ailments, including painful arthritis due to swollen joints, migraines, difficulty sleeping, difficulty staying asleep, a lack of energy, and brain fog that was so bad I actually went to my doctor, afraid I had early-onset dementia.

The bottom line as to why I felt so crappy and was constantly sick was because I wasn't giving my body the kind of nutrients it needed to work properly, so it simply couldn't get or stay healthy. It really was that simple, and I found that out after just a week of eliminating gluten from my diet. (I had done lots of research and asked a lot of health care professionals questions to help me figure out where to begin. This was what made sense for me. We will determine what your first step should be based on your particular needs.)

That one small change was eye-opening, so I added another by eliminating grains as well. Within a week of completely avoiding grains (which is not an easy task), I noticed that I had lost five pounds without even trying, my joints weren't quite as painful, and my brain fog didn't seem as bad as it had been. It was a real wake-up call and it motivated me to try another change – and when that made a difference, I tried another and another. *I became addicted to feeling good*, and when I brought my awareness to how I felt after every meal, I was able to identify things within my control that I could do to change my health. And when I ate foods that my body needed, I eliminated fatigue and found myself energized. Food was proving to be the absolute building block of everything. I could control what went into my mouth, so I could control much more of how I felt than I ever realized. That was empowering!

My husband, George, was witnessing first-hand the power of how changing a few of my eating habits was impacting my body and how my health was improving. He, too, began incorporating more awareness with his food choices and at the age of 58 is trim, fit, and playing ice hockey on a regular basis – and he's hotter than ever!

I've spent the last couple of years paying very close attention to the impact food has on how I feel, think, and function. I've also read everything I can to learn more about how and why food is such an important component in how we function because I now see the clear correlation. It comes down to the simple fact that food is the building block of every cell in your body, so doesn't it make sense that the quality of what you put into your body impacts the quality of your body and what it can do? Every cell in your body regenerates on a regular basis, so you are making new cells 24/7. If you use high quality materials (the foods that your body needs to perform at its most efficient and best self) then you're going to have a better quality of life. Period.

My list of symptoms and the foods that trigger them is long. I had no idea that the root cause of so many of the ailments that had plagued me for so long came down to each decision I made about what to eat. I didn't need to go on a particular diet, like Keto or low-fat. Instead, I needed to find out how *my* body reacted to everything from the types of food (dairy/meat/grain/etc.) to the quality (grass-fed/ organic/hormone, antibiotic free, processed, added sugars, etc.) I was consuming. Once I understood this information, I could then make choices as to what I wanted to do. If I wanted to eliminate the symptoms that were making me so sick I couldn't go to work and function any more, then I had to change my behaviors. If I wanted to continue down the path that I was on, which was pretty miserable at that point, then I could just continue eating the way I had been and I would have undoubtedly progressed even further on the unhealthy track I'd been on.

Society has made it super convenient for us to grab cheap and handy meals and snacks just about everywhere, but most of those options don't support the needs we have for sustained energy and stamina or to keep us at a healthy weight. We get so busy with jobs and other life events that our default mode often falls into picking up meals that are readily available even if they aren't serving our body's needs. The suggestions in this book will help you rebuild your gut, which is your "soil" from which everything else in your body is run. Once you get your gut in better shape, you'll feel the results throughout your entire body.

The most effective way I found of figuring out what worked for me was to deliberately monitor a specific food or food group and its impact on my health. When I finally came to this realization, it was hard to know where to start. I needed some kind of systematic way to learn which foods were possible culprits for my health issues so I could stop eating things that might be making me sick. I had to do a lot of research and visit a lot of professionals to come up with the information I needed in this process.

Once I compiled everything I learned about how food impacts our mental and physical health, I created the Mojo Meter as a way to assess my clients' biggest health challenges. The answers guide us to the strategies that will be most effective in helping them reach their goals. I based it on the process I used to figure out what I needed. Just like me, my clients need and expect to see results, and they need to see them fast. I had run out of patience and time for doing more of the same old treatments, and since the same old stuff wasn't working anyway, I finally realized they weren't going to work again, no matter how many times I repeated them. If I wanted different results, I needed to do something different. There was simply no getting around it.

I learned that the joint pain I'd experienced since I was a teenager wasn't actually a lifelong sentence – once I eliminated the foods that caused the excessive inflammation in my joints, I was addressing the root cause of the swelling, and I went from being dependent on anti-inflammatory drugs and pain medications and a cane to needing *no* medications and no longer hurting! Not only has the cane become a thing of the past, but because of my yoga practice, my body moves in ways it *never* has before (more on this part later).

There are a lot of resources out there with one-size-fits-all health plans and diets. Those don't take into consideration *your* particular health needs, environment, family, job, situation, and other variables. It's really hard to sift through everything and know what will work and what won't, but I will walk you through some resources I found to be particularly useful to help you discover what makes you function at your peak.

You are always *one decision away* from getting closer to your goal. You don't have to make a million decisions about how to change everything all at once. Just one decision at a time. Don't stress about your future decisions or what you will do tomorrow, just *focus on what you can do in this moment to change your momentum*. If you keep this principle in mind, you'll find this to be much more manageable and sustainable for the long haul, and isn't that your goal?

At first it felt like modifying my diet was all about "taking away" everything I loved. My comfort foods, the things I could make in a hurry, or meals I could pick up on my way home from work were ingrained in every aspect of what my family and I did, so making major changes that required a lot more thought, time, patience, and often money (yes, better quality food is more expensive than stuff that can be processed quickly and with inferior ingredients) was daunting, especially since I was tired and felt crappy. It wasn't long, however, before I noticed how powerful the tradeoff was – if I took the time to plan, prepare, and eat the types of foods that supported my brain and body, I became invincible. It was crazy amazing … and addicting. *It felt good* to have the weight melt off. It amazed me to see how quickly my skin cleared up, to the point where I often go out in public without make up on because I now feel so comfortable. The more attention I paid to what I was eating and how it made me feel, the more control I had in changing my destiny. That was empowering and I was hooked.

Now that you are ready to turn your health around, it's time to look at your results from your Mojo Meter so you can begin the transformation you desire and deserve. I can tell you about what I did to get healthy, but I can't do the work *for* you. I can do it *with* you and share the resources I used, and if you follow the advice in the book, you'll experience a freedom that comes with being well that changes your entire life. It becomes easier to do the things you have to do, and you find yourself feeling good enough to do the things you *want* to do (how long has it been since that's happened?). There will be challenges, but you will have the tools you need to overcome them. And if you want to jumpstart your wellness by checking out what else you can do, jump over to www.mPoweredEducator.com to connect with additional resources or reach out for more personal advice.

You won't be changing all your habits at once. Instead, you want to find the ones that will have the biggest and most positive impact. As you incorporate the changes prescribed for you based on the results of the first ten answers from your Mojo Meter, notice how you feel. Keep a journal that lets you see the connection between the food you are eating and the way your body responds. Then decide if you like those changes. If you do, great. If not, then make a different change.

You can refer back to the Mojo Meter and apply your specific results to find out how your meals can upgrade your life. For any of the questions to which you answered "true," I've indicated suggestions for which food groups you might want to consider eliminating for seven to ten days to see how your body reacts.

I was skeptical that food had anything to do with things like brain fog and arthritis pain, so I approached this with a suspicious but desperate mindset. Until I actually felt the incredible changes in my body, I hadn't believed the meals I ate could be that powerful and have such a powerful influence on every aspect of my mind and body. Boy, was I wrong!

Using the table below, find the area(s) that are the most troublesome for you. I've indicated which food groups could be causing or exacerbating your symptoms. If you have multiple questions to which you answered "true," find the food group that appears most for each of the questions and begin by eliminating that food group. That will help you address multiple symptoms at once – and the results will happen much faster and more effortlessly when you are hitting more than one area of your life.

I highly recommend keeping a food journal, even using an app to track what you're eating – I know you've heard it before and it's a drag, but it is an excellent tool for helping you see where you are making progress and where you still need help. It also makes it easier to make good food choices when you know you are holding yourself accountable in writing!

The food groups I suggest eliminating are based on research done from various medical practitioners, my personal nutritionist, the resources listed at the end of this book, and what I've learned through years of practice with my own body. Your body will react differently than anyone else's, so be sure to pay attention to how *you* feel. Write down not only what you eat, but how you feel before, during, and after your meals. A simple happy face, word, or other indicator is all you need to start seeing patterns in the relationship between your meals and how you feel.

The boxes that are blacked out indicate you should avoid or reduce your intake of those foods in order to identify if they are impacting you in a way that doesn't make you feel good.

mPower Method *Mojo Meter* for *Meals*:

STATEMENT	GRAINS OR AT LEAST GLUTEN	CARBS naturally found in foods	DAIRY	MEAT	SUGAR Added sugars & sweeteners
I have a lot of aches and pains.	■				
I often feel tired after eating.	■				■
My memory doesn't seem to be as sharp as it used to be.	■	■			
Other people have mentioned that I seem down or upset or not myself.	■	■			
I experience a lot of brain fog.	■	■			■
I don't have enough energy to get me through my days without it being a struggle.	■	■			
I experience digestive issues several times a week.			■		
I feel tired a lot of the time.	■				
I get a lot of illnesses, like colds, sinus infections, and other common and contagious ailments.	■		■		
I don't have any energy in reserve.	■				■
My weight is higher than what feels good.	■				
I experience frequent bloating.	■		■		
Sometimes I feel like all I want to do is cry and escape the exhaustion.	■				■

As you begin to make one change and then another, you'll be blown away by the results. By taking time each day to deliberately make choices about the meals you are using to fuel your brain and body, you are investing in a new and improved you, and that's why you are here in the first place.

In a nutshell, from what I've found in my own practice and with those with whom I work, there are some key food groups that have a huge impact across multiple areas you're trying to address. If you are struggling with weight, for example, your most effective way to address it is likely through the elimination of grains. Think about it – when farmers are fattening up their livestock, what do they feed them? Corn and other grains. Those grains do the same thing to your body that they do to the cows and pigs – they add weight and bulk you up. Don't believe me? See what happens if you eliminate grains from your meals for just one week. Not only will weight begin melting off, but you might also be delighted to discover that your brain fog is clearing up, along with the painful swelling of your joints. The benefits will become evident and you will quickly come to feel the correlation between what goes in your body and how you function.

By now, you may be a bit worried about what you *can* eat. It may seem like all I've focused on is elimination of food groups. That's because a huge part of getting and staying healthy is resetting your gut biome, and the only way to do that is to change what goes in your gut. But in addition to eliminating what isn't serving you well, you must also be vigilant about providing high quality meals that support brain and body health.

The list of what you can and should eat is long. For example, high quality lean meat serves to provide you with protein that's necessary for helping you function. Grass-fed beef and grass-fed dairy provide excellent sources of healthy fats that keep you going longer and at a steadier pace than any carbs and sugar can do. If you are not able to process or choose not to eat meat, your protein sources could include tofu, eggs, and nuts.

Many people turn to salads and other raw foods in an attempt to get healthy. Kale and other dark green veggies are full of vitamins, but if your body has difficulty processing them, they may cause you distress. Simply cooking them in a small amount of broth or high quality oil (olive, coconut, or avocado) for a few minutes to wilt them begins the digestion process and makes them gentler on your belly while still allowing you to access the nutritional benefits.

Action Plan:

Read each statement in the Mojo Meter for Meals. Select the one that is most problematic for you at this point. This is your starting place for your new meal modification plan.

- Write down the statement.

_____

_____

- What food group(s) is likely causing you this problem?

_____

_____

_____

- How will your life be better when the statement is no longer true? (For example, if your statement was "I have a lot of aches and pains," describe what you will be able to do and how you will feel when you no longer have to deal with those aches and pains.)

_____

_____

_____

_____

_____

• If you don't address this issue, how will it be impacting you in six months since you'll still be dealing with it? Is that okay with you?

_____

_____

_____

_____

_____

• What do you think will be the biggest hurdle for you in adapting to a new meal plan?

_____

_____

_____

_____

_____

• What is the reason you will strive to make this change, even when it's hard?

_____

_____

_____

_____

_____

- What will you do when it's hard to honor your decision?

  _____

  _____

  _____

  _____

  _____

  _____

Use a food journal or app on your phone to track your progress. Keep track of every food choice you make for the next twenty-one days. It takes that long to establish a new habit. And *notice how you feel* as your body adapts to the new changes. Sometimes the first few days our bodies actually feel worse before feeling better, so don't let that get you down. Just acknowledge it and know it will get better. Don't try to change everything at once – just the one thing you are focusing on at first.

Make a commitment to do your best to incorporate one new habit at a time *because you are investing in your well-being so you can regain your energy, health, and vitality.* You are worth it, so be as insistent on taking care of yourself as you would be if you were taking care of a loved one.

If you want to take your health to the next level, you may also want to explore the use of supplements and vitamins with your health care professional as those can provide immense support to your system in achieving and maintaining your health goals.

Chapter 6:

The mPower Method – Movement

"At first they will ask you why you're doing it.
Later they'll ask you how you did it."
–Anonymous

"**N**ow do a gentle swan dive to your forward fold," she said like it was an easy task. *Thud.* I wasn't even graceful when I fell flat on my face on the yoga mat. I was sweating like crazy, "downward dog" was pure agony, and every joint in my body was screaming at me to stop this awkward movement, but walking out would have been rude, so I stayed and finished the class. And for some reason, I went back the next day. But on the second day, I didn't fall over. I continued to sweat and the poses still seemed like I was trying to put my body into impossible pretzel shapes, but there was something about the gentle way this teacher invited the class to join her with movements that made our bodies feel good that made me want to experience this again and again.

I need to step back a moment and let you know that due to all kinds of problems relating to my skeletal system, I'd been advised to "take it easy" and not physically strain myself all my life. I've had reconstructive surgery on my back and neck. I have an artificial hip. I've had bunion removal. I spent five years in a back brace. I've had arthritis pain since I was a teenager. And the solution had always been to take it easy and take a pill. Well, this kind of yoga wasn't strenuous with impact, and it actually had components that made me feel good. And the last few minutes of each class ended with a pose called *savasana*, which is the time to lie on your back in corpse pose and let your body recalibrate after moving – essentially, it feels like a nap! What's not to love about that part?

The one part of yoga I knew wasn't for me involved slowing my mind down and focusing on my breath because, after all, I'm a busy woman with a thousand items on my to-do list. I didn't realize I was just the kind of person who would benefit from the very core principles of the yoga practice, nor did I realize how integral the training of the mind is in the success of *everything* else in life. So, in spite of fifty years of very little physical exertion and a million reasons why I couldn't exercise or quiet my mind, I decided it was worth a try because truly I had no other choice.

I started attending yoga classes at my local studio because it was convenient. It's only a mile and a half from my house, so I began walking to and from yoga. It was a nice way to breathe fresh air and be outside. I'll never forget my first class with Carrie, a somatic class. Somatic yoga is very gentle, so much so that I actually wondered if I was doing any kind of physical activity at all. At one point, we were lying on our backs with our feet to the floor. Carrie cued us to, "Gently roll your left foot to the knife's edge and then back to flat on the floor." Those seventeen words were game-changers for me. You see, for at least five years leading up to this point, I had to use my left hand to move my left leg in and out of the car, to cross it when I was seated, and any time I needed to move it independently. Yet when Carrie had us focus on the positioning of our feet, I found myself moving my leg (and artificial hip) effortlessly *and painlessly* for the first time in years! It was a lightbulb moment for me. Carrie had helped me focus my mind on what I *could* do, and then I could do more. Tears were rolling down my cheeks as I finally understood the potential for healing.

In order to function in a way that sustains you while also giving you the energy to move forward, you need to properly care for your body. There are no short cuts. No magic pills. No fancy creams. In short, if your body is going to *be* better, then you will have to actively do things that will help it *get and stay* better. For me, yoga provided the magic link I'd been missing in the movement part of my life.

It begins with gentle movement. Being mindful of what and how your body feels when you move it in certain ways will guide you toward what it needs. I was skeptical that the "exercise" that was called yoga wasn't aggressive enough or didn't make me work hard enough to lose weight, gain muscle tone, get rid of *all* my aches and pains, help me sleep better, reduce my stress level, and make my body and mind feel renewed and energized, but it sure as heck did!

The final few minutes of each yoga class pose, *savasana,* allows the body to recalibrate and process everything it did during the class. At first, my mind would race during this time. I could barely settle my body down because inevitably something would itch or muscles would twitch. Besides, how could being still be helping my body and mind? I wasn't *doing* anything, so how would I see improvement?

Here's a pretty important life-lesson – by *not* trying or doing, sometimes we can reach our goals in a manner that's more intuitive and more sustainable than when we work really hard. I wouldn't have believed it if I hadn't lived it because it goes completely against what society tells us about how we need to be faster, work harder, and do more. I've found the opposite to be true. For me, the practice of yoga pushed me harder than any "doing" exercise could have done. It invited me in to the gentle habits of noticing my breath, noticing how I felt, and noticing how I could use my breath and movement to ground me in every aspect of my life. It was a game-changer.

While yoga was what I found to be lifesaving, you may have the need for a different type of physical practice. The type of exercise isn't the important part. The important thing to remember is that regular movement is essential for your body to do what it was made to do. *Begin where you are* and move forward as your mind and body are ready. That may mean micro-movements or a non-impact activity like swimming, but whatever you choose, it's essential that you approach it not as another chore in your daily to-do list you have to get done, but instead as time you've set aside to care for yourself so you feel better. As I've said a million times, *notice how you feel* after you've done physical movement. And for heaven's sake, find a type of movement that makes you feel good. If you dread it, you won't do it.

Making changes that are successful is easier to do if you can see your progress. There are dozens of ways you can do this. For example, you could begin by using a pedometer and simply noticing if there is any correlation between the number of steps you take every day and something else, such as how well you sleep or whether your restless leg syndrome (RLS) is more manageable. The important thing is to do something different and then notice what is different in your outcomes.

Perhaps the thought of exercising makes you cringe. That's okay. Don't think of it as exercise. Rather it is through intentional movement that you are creating real, physical, permanent change for the better for yourself, so enjoy how good it feels. If you are doing something that doesn't feel good, then it isn't helpful to your mind or body, so find something else. Don't settle for something you can tolerate. Insist on finding something you'll crave because then you will make time for it and then you'll be successful in achieving your goals.

I have a couple of tricks I employ when movement seems to be too much:

- Listen to my body and rest. (Not every day, but sometimes this is as important as moving.)
- Fake it for five minutes. Do just five minutes of your favorite movement, then you can stop – if you want to. Which you probably won't, but if you do, that's okay.
- Listen to recordings (on YouTube or another platform) of hypnotist videos that are geared toward

motivating you to move or reach your goals. Just be present and listen.

- Phone a friend. See if someone wants to go for a walk, or go by yourself and just breathe fresh air and look around. You don't have to go fast or go far – but go outside.
- Find a playlist that gets you out of your funk or lets you dwell where you need to be and just escape with your headphones on and your eyes closed.
- Go outside. Be in nature. Sit in a chair and breathe the fresh air. No phone. No computer, No electronic devices. Maybe just a cup of tea. It can do wonders for rejuvenating you and making you feel like moving more.

When you are tired, the last thing you want to do is move. It seems like it's way too much effort. And even though you know that you'll end up with more energy after you move, that doesn't always translate into getting you off the couch and into some kind of movement. Just remember, our bodies were made to move. When we allow the joints to be used, they move more freely and without as much pain. When we get our heart rate elevated, blood moves to our extremities and energizes us. And when we keep our circulation going by engaging our bodies in movement throughout the day, germs don't settle in and make us sick. I'm living proof – and I used to be the *biggest* skeptic of exercise. Whether it's gardening, pole dancing, walking your dog, or some other kind of movement, just do it. Write it on your calendar and make it a priority. Look forward to it, knowing it's an investment in you!

Action Plan:

Identify the Movement Statement from the list below that is most true for you.

1. Look at the movement suggested for that statement.

2. Incorporate that movement (or something similar) into your routine at least four times a week. Write it in your calendar for the entire week: for example, write "walk thirty minutes" on your calendar for four times in the next seven days and then do it. The whole purpose is to get your body moving so there isn't stagnancy where disease can develop.

3. Keep a journal or use an app on your phone to track your progress.

   ○ A pedometer or other device that quantifies what you are doing can be helpful for noticing how the number of steps (or other activity you're measuring) impacts how you are feeling. That's the way to make the connection between your habits and your health, and that's how permanent change takes place!

4. Remember, it takes twenty-one days to establish a new habit, so give yourself time to make it feel like a natural part of your rhythm.

Movement Statements:

1. **I have not done much exercise in the past year.**
   Suggested movement: *yoga, swimming, walking, Tai Chi*

2. **I have physical limitations that prevent me from doing vigorous activities.**

Suggested movement: *yoga, swimming, walking*

3. **I prefer something with moderate physical activity.**
   Suggested movement: *jogging, Tae Kwon Do, Pilates, weight lifting*

4. **I prefer vigorous activities.**
   Suggested movement: *running, team sports, skiing, biking, Zumba, dance classes, spinning classes*

5. **I hate exercising.**
   Suggested movement: *team sports, horseback riding, aerobics, or another activity where you are focused on something besides the actual movement*

Remember: if you don't do something different, you won't get different results. It's time to make permanent positive changes for *you*!

Chapter 7:

The mPower Method – Music

"So long as the human spirit thrives on this planet,
music in some living form will sustain
and accompany it."
– Aaron Copland

E verything in the universe vibrates. Everything. The cells in your body and every square inch of the wreckage of the Titanic at the bottom of the ocean are full of atoms and molecules that are bouncing around constantly. Sound waves travel through the air and water and bounce off of us and everything in its path. Our bodies respond to the vibrations of music, and the way our bodies respond to the vibrations around us directly impacts how we feel. (I won't bore you with any more science-y stuff, but this is important to remember.)

Think about it: your mind and body feel very different when you are singing *Silent Night* in a candle lit church on

Christmas Eve than when you're in a bar where there's loud music booming from the subwoofers and everyone is singing and dancing. In the first instance, you might feel relaxed, nostalgic, and perhaps even peaceful. Those are very real emotions and they have physical traits such as feeling calm and safe and having a reduced heart rate. Your breathing would likely be slow and deep. Yet if you were at that bar with the booming music, you'd physically feel the vibrations throughout your body to the point where you'd likely be moving to the beat either consciously or subconsciously, and your heart rate would respond, as would many of your other behaviors. You'd be likely to engage in activities that involve heavy food and alcohol and dancing, whereas if you were in the first setting, you'd be more likely to act in a more mindful and careful manner.

The music in any given circumstance impacts how you feel and therefore how you think and what you do. We are manipulated by music *all* the time. Think about the grocery store, mall, commercials, car radio, and everything else you encounter on a daily basis. There seems to always be music playing, and in many cases, the music is selected to invoke a particular behavior that often results in a financial profit for the provider of the music. It's that powerful.

Music has the power to heal. It can make you feel emotions. It causes your brain to function differently. And it reaches across cultures, gender, and other barriers. Whether you consume music by playing recordings you like or create your own music as a musician, it is an essential part of being healthy. Think of music as another tool you can use on your journey to the new you!

In addition to using music in traditional ways to help manage emotions or motivate you to do physical movement, there are other healing ways the vibrations of musical tones can impact your health.

Tibetan singing bowls are an example of how the use of tones with harmonic overtones can be used to reset and calibrate the human body and help it heal. I first had the experience of a "sound bath" shortly after falling in love with yoga. One of my former students, Kim, was offering this at a yoga studio, so my husband and I checked it out. For ninety minutes, we laid on our backs, cozy on our mats, while Kim played these beautiful bowls. The vibrations of some of the bowls resonated deep within my spine, and the overtones could be felt sympathetically elsewhere in my body. I wasn't just hearing the sound with my ears – I was *feeling the sound in my body.* Once I felt those vibrations, I was energized yet calmed. It was beautiful. It was so powerful, in fact, that I invited her into my classroom where she shared this experience with all my students, 60 kids an hour for an entire school day. The students were intrigued and the feedback I got from them was very positive. They are attuned to vibrations all the time when we are playing music (that's all music is, after all), and this kind of awareness within their bodies was a new dimension to help them *feel* the music differently.

Bringing an awareness to how our bodies respond to the vibration of music allows us to use music to change how our bodies and minds feel. Don't believe me? Put on a song from your teenage years and close your eyes. Are you transported back in time? Are you feeling feelings you experienced when you were that age? Do you notice how your body reacts when you feel those familiar vibrational patterns? Music is *that* powerful, so use it to your advantage to help you heal and stay healthy.

Music can be very personal, and this is where I'd encourage you to think about ways you want to incorporate music in your healing journey. Here are a few ideas, but the possibilities are endless.

Music can be used to support the other components of the mPower Method. Create playlists or opportunities to listen to or perform music that enhances your ability to meet your goals. Here are some ideas of how music can be a powerful tool in your emotional and physical healing.

- **Meal music:** If you find yourself eating too fast, create a playlist that consists of music that calms you. Pay attention to the music as you prepare and eat your meals, taking full advantage of the atmosphere, emotions, and feelings that come to you from the music and enjoy your meals at the pace dictated by your playlist.

- **Movement music:** When you need to get moving, music can make it happen faster than just about anything else. Find the tunes that get your blood pumping, heart racing, and body grooving to the beat and let them help you get going on your walk or jog. Or if you've had a crazy-busy day (and who hasn't?), then have a playlist of music that calms you as you do gentle stretching and other yoga type movements.

- **Restorative music:** Playlists aren't just for music, movement, and meals. You can use music to help you study, sleep, calm down, feel energized, experience melancholy, feel happy, and so much more. Begin noticing how your body reacts to different kinds of music. What music makes you feel like moving a little more? What music makes you sleepy? Use those answers to your advantage and incorporate the opportunities for combining music with movement, meals, and mindfulness to get the most out of your transformation. I've had clients who find hypnotist videos to be extremely helpful as they want to focus on improving study skills, being more creative, and sleeping better. The music and use of various sounds (such as brain wave patterns) enhance their experiences at whatever they are looking to improve.

- **Playing music**: If you are a musician, or if you would like to become a musician, seek out opportunities to play your own music. It's a creative outlet, lets you express emotions, gets you working with others, and creates bonding opportunities with other people as you practice and play together.

Action Plan:

You are going to create a playlist to help you achieve your goals.

Looking at the categories above, select the one area you feel music will have the biggest impact on, supporting you the most at this time.

If you are struggling with falling or staying sleep, for example, perhaps you'll begin with a Restorative playlist. Look at the music on your devices and see what you already have that can help put you in a calm mood for sleep. One of the best resources is hypnotist and mindfulness videos that help you put yourself in the proper head space for restorative sleep. Likewise, there are videos and music to support you if you need energy, creativity, or any other kind of motivation.

What category are you going to focus on first?

Check out YouTube, Spotify, and other media playlists to find selections that you can use when you want music to energize, calm, motivate, or bring out other emotions. There are endless options, and you can also create your own personalized playlists with all your favorites. In this day and age of technology, you have access to more music than you'll ever need, so take advantage of it and allow it to be part of your health plan.

Those are just a few examples. You know your taste in music and how your mind and body react to what you hear, so build playlists to your advantage and use them. This is a no- to low-cost way to make all of the other components of the mPower Method work even better.

Chapter 8:

The mPower Method – Mindfulness

"Being healthy means having
a healthy body and a healthy mind.
If you can keep your mind healthy,
you will help the health of your body."
– Virginia Madsen

This is the chapter where you learn how to make this transformation work for the long-term. You already know what doesn't work and that's why you're here right now, so you don't need to waste any more time, money, or energy on fad diets, prescriptions that have worse side effects than the original symptoms for which they were pre-scribed, or anything else that doesn't serve you. What you *do* have to do, however, is learn how to make changes that stick.

We have been programmed through millions of years of evolution to first and foremost survive. Congratulations. You woke up today. Life is tough, but you're tougher.

You've survived everything else in your life so far, so your subconscious is going to do everything in its power to repeat stuff you've already done and lived through in order to up your chances of making it another day. But we both know that repeating more of the same actions will only get you more of the same feelings and results you've been experiencing. You are reading this because you realize that's not working for you, so I know you are ready for the work that is ahead.

In Chapter 9, you will find my SNaP Strategies, simple steps you can begin practicing immediately to learn how to be more mindful of what you are experiencing. Incorporating a new SNaP strategy is a practice of drawing your awareness to something you've been doing on auto-pilot it becomes a new experience. It's only when we are aware of something that we can change it. There is power in awareness!

Author Jack Canfield said, "When people start focusing on what they want, what they don't want falls away, and what they want expands, and the other part disappears." This is the core of the basis of the mPower Method: being mindful. Deepak Chopra's book *Leadership of the Soul* is full of wisdom. One of my favorite nuggets has been at the core of this whole journey: "That's the nature of habit, to reappear on its own."

It's time for you to create new habits. To *be* the person you want to be – now. Don't wait until you feel like you deserve to be that person. Act like her this very moment. What would she do? What kinds of decisions will she make when she is at her peak and wants to remain there? Make those choices *today* and you become her … today!

Toxic stress impairs attention, emotion and mood regulation, sleep, learning, productivity, creativity, and many more areas of our life. What we often forget is that stress also has a huge impact on our physical and mental health. If you only read and follow the advice in one chapter of the book, this is the one to do because a mindfulness approach to life is a game-changer in every other aspect of your life.

Let's go back to early 2017, when I was at my lowest point. I was having all kinds of physical symptoms that kept sending me from one specialist to the next. The digestion issues (constant feeling of nausea and unsettled gut), memory problems, arthritis, hormonal imbalances, and everything else were being looked at as independent ailments with independent solutions that usually consisted of more pills. What I was doing was trying to mask symptoms so I could get on with all the things I had to do so as to not let anyone down (sound familiar?). It was only when I began to *notice how I was feeling* and what circumstances contributed to those feelings that I could approach my health care in a way that made sustainable changes.

Noticing how I was feeling was more than identifying what part of my body hurt, it also meant noticing how I felt in relation to what I had done. For example, if my stomach was feeling particularly nauseous, I needed to identify what I had been eating so I could look for patterns and take different action if what I was doing wasn't working. I needed to become aware of how my behaviors were impacting my health; otherwise, I couldn't do anything to change them. Being mindful and observing my actions and what happened as a result of my actions marked the pivotal point in turning me around from over 30 years of health issues that had accumulated and left me a toxic mess.

Now it's your turn. It's time for you to give yourself the same loving attention and care you've been giving to everyone else for years and years. This process isn't an instant fix, but you will begin receiving benefits immediately – and if you are mindful, you will notice those benefits. It's kind of like an addiction once you experience how one then two then three small changes begin to make you feel.

What is mindfulness? In a nutshell, it's simply *being fully present in the here and now.* That's it. Sounds simple, doesn't it? But it's anything but simple in this fast-paced, over-stimulating, hyper-crazy world in which we live. Everything and everyone is telling us that we need to be more productive, buy more stuff, have faster electronic devices, constantly be connected via social media, and the list goes on. It's exhausting. And every interaction or action you take where your mind and body are being stressed (and by the way, stress happens even when you are doing things you love) causes your body to send out cortisol, the stress hormone, which is meant to save you in a fight-or-flight situation (like being chased by a tiger). In short-term situations, this can be a lifesaver at best, and it also serves to help get things done in a hurry.

But the reason you are reading this book right now is because you've discovered that your body is shooting out that cortisol *way* too much. How do you know? You can see and feel it in your mind and body. Perhaps it shows up as brain fog, arthritis, chronic illnesses, constant catching of colds and other infections, feeling overwhelmed, being too tired to sleep, lacking energy, and being exhausted. Your body is being bombarded by hormones that are meant to be used only during times of stress, so it's sending you into chronic stress and you are suffering from the miserable effects. That can end now, and you can make it happen.

There are some steps you can take and routines you can establish to change the path on which you are currently traveling. If your current situation isn't serving you, then why do you continue repeating the same awful feelings day after day? If you don't change something, nothing changes, and that's no longer acceptable to you. You are ready to make changes that support the lifestyle you've worked so hard to create. Change is uncomfortable. Nature protects us as a species by programming our brains to stay alive. Your brain wakes up each day and thinks, "What I did yesterday didn't kill me, so I'll repeat the same stuff and I'll survive another day." Its purpose is to keep you alive, but are you really thriving or just surviving?

Once I discovered the personal benefits of a mindfulness practice, I knew I had to share the practice with my students. They, too, were experiencing signs of stress that were unhealthy. The constant stimulation, social media, peer and parent pressure, and so much more had them in a frenzy. As amazing and mature as high school band kids are, they are nonetheless teenagers, and for every hour of every single day of my career for thirty-one years I have had a group of forty to seventy-five kids walk into my classroom, get their instruments out, and make music. That encompasses a lot of energy!

Even though the students in my classes remain pretty constant throughout the year, from day to day each of them has life experiences that cause them to grow, so the makeup of each class from day to day changes just a little. Their needs vary based on external and internal stimuli. Some of them lead fairly easy lives with supportive parents and very little to worry about while others come from broken homes, have to work to help pay bills, and may be in transitional housing. Yet they come into my classroom with the expectation of learning to play beautiful music with one another. For years, I'd settle them down by playing scales and other warm up routines. Then I introduced breathing exercises to expand our lung capacities before playing. Yet I never felt completely grounded, and that made it hard to help them feel grounded and truly focus on the task at hand.

Enter a mindfulness practice.

From the time I missed school in March of 2017 until I returned to work the following September, they could see something drastic had happened. I had lost quite a bit of weight in just a few months (and with it a lot of the illnesses and physical pain that went along with the extra weight) and was much more centered. Not only was I thinner, but my skin had cleared up and kids told me I "just seemed different." I explained the health issues I'd gone through and that my healing had taken place as a result of me taking care of my mental as well as my physical health. I told them that when they came into class every day and we got ready to start, it always felt like we were in a snow globe, with lots of energy buzzing around us. The energy wasn't necessarily a bad thing, but with all of us coming into the room with our own life experiences impacting our mood and physical well-being, it was only natural that it took a lot of work to stay focused and on-task. (Something the kids did quite well, I might add, but it took constant effort.) Once I applied a mindfulness practice to my own life and learned the benefits of being grounded before doing things, I saw a 180-degree turnaround in my health. If it was that powerful for me, I imagined it could be as powerful for the kids.

If the beginning of each class felt like we were in a snow globe that was being shaken up, then my mind often felt like it was constantly in that state – only ten times worse! When I began doing yoga and learning to slow down my mind and be present in the moment, I noticed that the snow globe effect was calming down inside me. Over the course of a month or two, I started learning to observe and release many of the thoughts that were whirling around in my head rather than judging them or being sucked into worrying about them, and it was freeing. What if I tried that with my students at the beginning of each class? Could we in effect take all of our unbridled energy and settle it down, get grounded, and recalibrate ourselves to a common frequency upon which we could then begin our learning each day? That was the million-dollar question – and after a year and a half of daily practice of this with my classes, the answer is a resounding *heck yeah*! If a bunch of teenagers can do this, then so can you.

I have to admit that when I first introduced this to the students, there were some skeptics. I created a five-minute routine that includes guided breathing and relaxation and ends with us playing our warm up chorale. It felt a little odd to many of them to be asked to close their eyes and do a mindfulness practice while surrounded by their peers. But they are amazing young men and women and they did what I asked, even if it made them think I'd lost my marbles for a while. We've spent a lot of time talking about and reflecting on how this mindfulness practice has impacted them as individuals and us as ensembles. Their insight has been enlightening. They've told me how they've used this technique to relax before tests, to sleep, to help them study, to deal with grief, and so much more. They have articulated how the classroom experience is more focused and productive because we take the time to get settled each day before starting class. They've seen how it helps me serve them better.

In the beginning, there were days when I questioned if it was really making a difference (and you will do that, too) but I want to encourage you to never let go of hope. One day you will look back and see how it has all come together; what you have wished for has come to be and you'll be able to look back, laugh, and ask yourself how the heck you managed to get through all of that. Change is a process, so be patient with yourself and make the commitment that you owe yourself the peace of mind and health to live the life you worked so hard to create. When you slip up, acknowledge it, and let it go. Move on. Whatever happened is over. Let it go. I say that like it's easy to do. It's not. It takes practice. And it takes determination to see it through if you are going to see results. If you want different results, you must do things differently. If you don't, your life will not be different. And you are here right now because you are desperate for change. So let's keep going.

As you begin to practice mindfulness, you'll discover it is time to let some things go, simply for the reason that they are heavy. You can come up with a million reasons why you think you need to continue doing the very things that got you here in the first place, and as long as you argue for your limitations, you get to keep them. You will be stuck and unable to move forward. *Or*, you can slow down (even though you are convinced you don't have time to do just that), find your breath, and get grounded.

Just like a snow globe that's been shaken up, it takes time for your mind and body to settle down. If you try to get the snow globe to settle down while you're still holding it and carrying on with your regular activities, the snow may fall slower, but it won't completely stop and allow you to see the objects in the snow globe. You must allow it to be completely still long enough for the water to stop swirling and the glitter to follow the pull of gravity and settle on the bottom. It only takes a matter of minutes until it settles, revealing the magical scene inside, and the very glitter that was covering up the view when it was moving around has become a lovely blanket of snow that grounds the scene in the snow globe. But without a few minutes of stillness, it is impossible for it to become completely settled. So it goes with a mindfulness practice. Your mind and body need time to go from hyper-speed to a pace that serves you well, a place where you have space to think – and space to *not* think. That begins by bringing stillness to your body and to your mind. Easy to say – hard to do … until you practice it every day and it becomes habit.

As I've learned through the use of this practice in my personal life and classroom implementation of this technique, recalibrating the mind and body makes us more ready for the three R's of learning: *receiving* input, *retaining* information, and *responding* with the knowledge in new and innovative ways.

Whether you prefer using mindfulness strategies through the practice of yoga, meditation, or other means is not relevant. It's the actual practice of being mindful of what is happening in the present moment, how your mind and body are responding to stimuli, and how you feel that allow you to be in touch with your environment and inner self in a way that has to be experienced to be understood. And once you discover it, you'll wonder how you ever survived without being grounded.

On my website, mPoweredEducator.com, you can find videos with meditations to help you get centered. If you use them (or other meditation practices) daily, you will find yourself quickly learning how to put yourself in a state of mind and body where you are able to be focused, calm, and ready to function at your peak. It takes a little practice, but I promise that if you take ten minutes a day for twenty-one days, you'll experience true transformation – and you will be hooked because there's no limit to where you can go.

Action Plan:

You are going to learn how to draw your attention to what you are doing in the present moment. This is a game-changer, so embrace the opportunity to experience every aspect of your life in a completely new way. It takes practice and is much harder to do than it seems like it should be. Don't beat yourself up when you find your mind wandering. Simply acknowledge the distraction and bring your attention back to the task at hand.

The action plan for this chapter is to go on to the next chapter where we will explore SNaP Strategies, which are like mini-training exercises to teach you to be mindful. At the end of Chapter 9, the action plan outlines what to do as it applies to the Mindfulness segment of the mPower Method.

Write down your observations in a journal or the notes section of your phone or wherever else makes sense for you. Those notes become a very valuable tool in seeing and identifying the progress you are making. You want to celebrate each step because that's what gives you the incentive to keep going on this journey when things get difficult, and those milestones are easier to recognize when you've taken the time to articulate them and can look back at how far you have come.

Chapter 9:

SNaP Strategies – Start Now and Progress (SNaP)

"If you want to change your life,
first change your mindset.
You can't find opportunity
when you are looking for excuses."
– Anon

I n this chapter is a list of SNaP Strategies. It consists of many ideas you can use to train yourself to be mindful. Some of them may seem silly or irrelevant, but if you trust me and play along, you will find that bringing your awareness to something as mundane as how you brush your teeth will cause you to look at everything else through a different filter. It's the key element to becoming mindful.

Quitting a bad habit is impossible by itself. Replacing that bad habit with a different habit is very doable. That's how you make significant and real change. If all you do is focus on what you are giving up, you'll feel empty. Instead, the key is to practice replacing habits you don't even realize you have with free and easy small changes so you can see what happens when you bring awareness to what you are doing.

Read through the SNaP Strategies. Find one, two, or three that seem doable and make a commitment to be mindful of that behavior every time you are in the situation and just notice how it makes you feel.

Start Now and Progress*
* SNaP Strategies to jump-start your transformation
Categories:
Weight / **I**nsomnia / **A**ches and Pains / **S**tress / **E**xhaustion

If you have specific issues you want to address, such as weight, insomnia, etc., then select actions that are indicated in parenthesis as focusing on those areas.

- Record your heart rate before and after doing a short meditation video of your choice. Begin to notice how you feel after doing this for a week. If your heart rate is lower after the meditation or you feel calmer, you might want to consider continuing this practice. If you have an app for tracking this data, look at it and see how your body is responding to the mindfulness relaxations. (S / I)
- Change your alarm sound to something soothing rather than the horrific fire-truck-plowing-through-your-bedroom-wall sound that currently jars you out of your sleep every morning. (S)

- Brush your teeth with your non-dominant hand. (S)
- Color. Draw. Paint. Doodle. Create. (S / A)
- Play music. (S / A / E / W / I)
- Sit at a different chair when you eat dinner. (W / S)
- Chew each bite thirty or more times. (W / A / S)
- Put your fork down between every bite. Don't pick it up until you are ready to eat the next bite. (W / A / S)
- Part your hair differently. (S)
- Take a "stay-cation" by spending the night in another room of your own home. Approach it like it's a hotel or getaway cottage and look at it with fresh eyes. (I / A / S / E)
- Take a different route to work. (S / W)
- Change your passwords to a positive phrase or a goal you have to remind yourself of what's important to you every time you type them. (S / W)
- Move your trash can to the other side of your sink. (S)
- Take a break from social media (you'll be glad you did!). (S!!! / W / I / A / E)
- Eat with your non-dominant hand. (Added bonus – helps with weight loss!) (W / S)
- Listen to a hypnotist video on YouTube. (There are hundreds of different videos that can help you with everything from falling asleep to being focused and alert.) Select videos that are geared toward your particular wants and needs. (S / W / I / A / E)
- Seek out opportunities to compliment others. (S / E)
- Allow someone to go ahead of you in line at the store. (S)

- Set your alarm for nine minutes earlier. Use those nine minutes to visualize your day going exactly how you want it to go before you do your normal routine. How do you feel when you picture different parts of your day turning out the way *you* want them to? (S / E / A / W)
- Set your alarm for nine minutes earlier and use those nine minutes to listen to an inspiring song, spend time in meditation, or having a cup of tea with your cat. Whatever makes you happy, just do it. (S / W / E / A)
- Avoid electronic devices for the first hour of your day. (S / W / A)
- Pay it forward next time you buy coffee. (S)
- Light a candle while you get ready for work. (S / E / A)
- Listen to a different radio station (or watch a different news channel) or avoid the news altogether for a while. (S / A / I / W / E)
- Based on the results of your Mojo Meter assessment, select one thing to change this week. Notice all the ways that decision makes you feel, then you can decide if you want to continue with the new habit going forward. For example, if you gave up beverages with added sugar because you wanted to get rid of the jitters, you might also note that you lost three pounds, weren't so cranky, your skin cleared up, and you didn't have afternoon sugar crashes. After looking at all the benefits from just giving up your sugar-laced beverages, you will probably find that a small price to pay for all those feel-good changes, so

the decision to limit those kinds of drinks becomes simple. If you didn't like the changes you saw from the habit you tried, then there's no need to continue with the new habit. (W / I / A / S / E)

- Try an online yoga or other class that involves gentle movement. (W / A / I / S / E)
- Add a cup of tea to your morning routine – and enjoy it while you do nothing at all but simply sit and drink it. No phone. No TV. No distractions. Just enjoy a cup of tea. Use a lovely mug. Sit somewhere peaceful. Notice how it smells, tastes, and makes you feel as it warms you from the inside out. (W / A / S / E)
- Turn off the notifications on your phone. Do you really need to be interrupted constantly with trivial stuff? (S / I / E)
- Put your phone on Do Not Disturb 24/7. You'll survive. You can set it so family and anyone else you want are still able to reach you, but cut down on the constant interruptions by choosing when to be on the phone or return text messages. (S / I / E / W / A)
- If you wear a Fitbit or other device that buzzes you when you get notifications, turn that off, too. The constant distractions make it impossible to get into flow for anything. (S / A / E / I / W)

For example, you might pick brushing your teeth with your non-dominant hand as your first SNaP awareness exercise. You'll only do this a couple times a day, but it will become a new experience when you are doing it in a different way. First of all, when you open the cabinet to get your toothbrush, bring awareness as to which hand automatically reached for it, then use the other one. Apply the toothpaste using the opposite hand you normally use to squeeze the tube. How does that change things? Before putting the toothbrush in your mouth, notice what your mouth, teeth, and tongue feel like, taste like, and even smell like. And when you brush, really notice how the pressure of the toothbrush feels on your teeth, gums, cheeks, and tongue. What does your toothpaste taste like? Is it refreshing and does it wake up your mouth? Is there any kind of texture to it? How does your body let you know it's time to spit rather than swallow the toothpaste? What kinds of signals does it send? And how do your tongue, teeth, and mouth feel after a thorough brushing? Just be aware. You've brushed your teeth every day for most of your life, but have you ever *really* paid attention to what it feels like? Did this change your experience?

Or maybe you are in a rut, which often leads to insomnia, exhaustion, aches and pains, and other maladies. While a vacation would be nice, that's not always an option when you need to recharge. But could you have a stay-cation in your own home? What if you spruced up your guest room and spent the night there? You wouldn't have to pack a suitcase or spend money, but the simple change of scenery and experiencing your house in a new way can be very eye-opening. You might be able to relax in a space where you haven't been conditioned to stay awake at night and worry. Perhaps you could close the door and enjoy a cup of tea, read a book, or even take a nap. You'd be surprised how this can serve as a great way to get a new perspective or break a bad habit (especially if you don't have a TV in the guest room!).

At first you may have a hard time making a connection between how activities like this can improve your aches and pains or help you cope with stress, but what I've learned over decades of study and practice is that when we engage in meaningful activities, it has a positive impact on *every* aspect of our lives. You might wonder how putting your phone on Do Not Disturb will impact your weight, but if you *really* think about it, are there times when a call or text or other notification triggers an emotion that leads to unhealthy behaviors like stress-eating or drinking or robbing you from the ability to be present in the here and now because your thoughts got pulled into whatever latest notification popped up? Or perhaps you mindlessly graze while being distracted with other activities, so you don't even enjoy the calories you consume.

Practicing these strategies simply opens the door for you to figure out other ways you can bring more purpose to your actions. You'll think of other habits or ideas you want to incorporate, so don't be afraid to embrace them. The point is to bring awareness to what you are doing rather than just going through life on auto-pilot.

If you aren't sure where to begin, pick a category where you want to experience a jump-start to change and try ideas for your specific goals. Whatever you do, bring your total awareness to *everything* surrounding the change(s) you are making. Be fully present in the experience in the same kind of detail I explained with the example above with brushing your teeth. What have you got to lose? Seriously. You've come this far, so why not take the next step?

Incorporating one or a few of these strategies into your daily routine can help you discover the types of actions you can take to impact you in positive ways. You might find you are able to be more focused at work if your phone notifications aren't buzzing on your Fitbit all day. Or that when you replace a Diet Coke with unsweetened tea in the afternoon, you eliminate your afternoon headaches. A lot of this is trial and error, but doing nothing is only error, so what have you got to lose? Remember, it's being mindful of how your choices make you feel that is key to making lasting changes.

Chapter 10:

The mPower Method – Putting It All Together

"In Japan, broken objects are often repaired with gold. The flaw is seen as a unique piece of the object's history, which adds to its beauty. Consider this when you feel broken."
– Humanity's Team

When I began writing this book, I thought it would have all the answers about how to go back to work and never get sick again, because I was doing a really good job at not getting those pesky illnesses anymore. But writing the book was just the beginning of discovering much more than just how to "not get sick." It allowed me to really evaluate where I was in my health and professional journeys and helped me make choices to support the healing that had taken place over the course of the previous year and a half. This process also opened my eyes to how I needed to be mindful of not putting unreasonable stress on my mind and body by working in a new way that made my healthier lifestyle sustainable.

So many positive changes occurred in my body and brain in the first several months of my transformation. My arthritis pain had ceased. I no longer had migraines. My weight was down to what it had been when I graduated from high school over thirty-five years before. My ADHD symptoms were manageable most of the time. I was able to sleep and I actually felt good, plus, I was off all the pharmaceuticals I'd been on for decades. I managed to put some reasonable boundaries up that allowed me to keep my work and family lives relatively separated for the first time in my entire career. I thought I could keep going at this pace.

But I was wrong. It's through this writing process that I realized I needed to take my own advice and get to the root cause of my illness. In spite of all the health gains I'd made, I continued to deal with relentless nausea and food aversions that keep me from being able to hold down food much of the time. A chronic issue with my adrenal glands mean there are days that go by where I am unable to eat anything at all, making it unbelievably hard to function as a teacher who has up to 75 kids an hour with whom I am constantly interacting. By the time I'd taught the first three hours of the day, I'd been responsible for over 175 teenagers and my energy reserves had been depleted, and I still had nearly 100 more kids to go before my instructional duties ended for the day and then the inevitable afternoon and evening meetings, performances, and sporting events would begin.

Even though I had been practicing mindfulness for eighteen months at this point and had made so much progress in so many aspects of my health recovery, this was a losing battle. I'd get to the point where I couldn't physically focus on the computer monitor or make decisions because there was nothing to fuel my body and brain. Standing in front of a classroom full of teenagers and teaching hour after hour while making decisions and having my sympathetic nervous system constantly bombarded by noise and other stimulation was becoming increasingly impossible when I wasn't getting the nutrition my brain and body needed to do all the executive functioning required of my job.

How I could write a book when I couldn't even figure this out for myself, I wondered. So I reread the parts I already wrote and then I took my own (fantastic) advice – *I must be mindful of what my body is telling me. If I don't listen to the subtle messages, something worse will have to happen to get my attention, and I can't afford to hit rock bottom again.*

I wanted to be back at the job I love so dearly, but once again the physical toll on my body was becoming harder to ignore, so I had to be mindful of what I needed to do to protect my job and my health.

And then I realized the answer to getting back to work without getting sick again meant doing *whatever it takes* to protect my health and my job (in that order). This was something I'd known in my heart of hearts for a long time, but I hadn't been willing to admit that I was no longer (and maybe never was) able to handle the demands of my job at the level I'd been trying to maintain for so many years. It took me a long time to say the words out loud, but once I heard myself acknowledge how unbelievably hard this has been on me and the toll it's taken on my mental and physical health, then I finally knew what I had to do. I needed to look at the options I had that would reduce the strain on my body so I could get to the root cause of what was causing the unrelenting nausea, even if that meant modifying my responsibilities at work.

After consulting with my doctors and trying every type of solution recommended from physicians and other health experts, a reduced workload became the only option. The mere thought of reducing my paycheck this close to retirement while we still had college loans for three kids to finish paying off, a mortgage, and a hundred other reasons why this didn't make any sense seemed like the worst idea ever, until I considered the alternative. How many more times would my body bounce back if I continued to ignore the screaming it was doing at me? I'd had too many close calls in the past that landed me in the hospital and on sick leave for months at a time, so I figured my odds were not improving when it comes to recovering if I get super sick again.

It was time to be mindful of the cost if I were to continue to push through at this pace – and this time I wanted the outcome to be different, so I had to listen to my body and the advice of people who are a lot smarter than I am. I accepted a six-week reduced work schedule so I could continue to serve my students (which fills my soul), earn a portion of my paycheck, and continue to search out a root cause for my health issue.

"What if you feel better after reducing your schedule? Then what?" my husband asked. I think his real worry was that we'd find that my health would improve when I wasn't working full time and that would mean a permanent reduction in our family's income. That was scary to think about, but so was the prospect of being so sick I couldn't eat and knowing I could only go so long without fuel in my body before I'd crash even harder. The vicious cycle reared its ugly head again, even after I had conquered so many other health issues.

And then it hit me: life is a journey. Things happen. We must learn to adjust. I had been so rigid for thirty-one years in my career that I couldn't imagine success as doing any other job or doing it in any other way than to put my heart and soul into it at all costs, and *that* had been the real problem. I was only measuring success by whether or not I could return to work in the same capacity as before. I'd already had plenty of proof that that wasn't sustainable, yet I didn't want to hear that message. So once again, my body was rebelling.

The true conflict in my life had been between my love for my job and wanting to be the best high school band director on the planet while also wanting to be the best mom and wife and everything else I thought I had to be. There was a cost to this pursuit. The price I paid was my chronic health issues that made everything seem so much harder. I had to come up with a way to sustain the lifestyle I'd chosen.

The components of meals, movement, and music are incredibly important contributors to quality of life, but the most critical component of the mPower Method is mindfulness, the ability to bring awareness to relationships between what you do and how you feel. Once you consciously recognize those relationships, you can begin to change them, letting go of that which doesn't serve you and doing more of what does.

I am continually reminded of this important connection between being aware of the impact my choices of what I eat, how I move, and what I listen to have on how I ultimately feel. Every single time I bring my awareness to the outcome of my choice (for example, how I will feel if I eat pasta), the decision becomes clear. I know pasta (thanks to the gluten) makes me feel very sick to my stomach, tired, and gives me brain fog. I hate feeling that way, so suddenly eating pasta is no longer a viable option for me. That is the power of mindfulness.

You may be in a place where you have to make a major choice or change you didn't plan on making, at least not yet. Maybe retirement is on the horizon, but you can't afford it for a few more years, so you need a plan, one that will allow you to get back to work without getting sick again. Finding sustainable ways in which you can return to work and still find a manageable balance between your professional life and your personal life might require you to think outside the box.

I always assumed I would teach high school band up until the day I retired – and by "retired," I was thinking that meant stopping work for good and being able to live on my pension. I figured that would be when I turned sixty-five. I really thought I could and should continue at this break-neck pace, making work the center of everything I do. But that wasn't and isn't healthy. It took me long enough to figure it out, and it took me even longer to admit it to myself, but once I did, I discovered the possibilities of creating a sustainable and manageable future that included a healthy balance of the type of work that I can do given where I am at this stage in my life.

We all have some kind of chronic issue that challenges us. Maybe it's our personal health. Maybe it's a parent for whom we are caring, or a child with special needs, or a partner who isn't home very often. The key to success isn't in eliminating all causes of stress. It's learning how to respond, not react, to the stressors that show up in your life and making decisions that help you be the best version of you that you can be!

I started with baby steps – reducing my workday by two classes (thus reducing my student-load by nearly one hundred kids per day). Doing that meant exhausting my sick leave and looking at other options for income, but it allowed me to be fully present when I was teaching. What I found as the result of this journey is that in order for me to be the best teacher I could be without running myself into the ground, I had to reevaluate my definition of "returning to work." I became obsessed with figuring this out for myself, and in the process, I became even more obsessed with helping other women find their own life balance who are in this same downward spiral that is sucking the life out of them to find.

If you have been missing work or dragging through each day only to return to the same job with the same stressors and you end up in the cycle of getting healthy, getting sick, missing work, going back, etc., then perhaps you, too, need to look at how you can meet your professional goals, financial needs, and personal growth in ways that support your mental and physical health.

Before you shake your head and think *she can't possibly understand my situation and how it wouldn't be possible for me to reduce my hours or find a new job*, know that at the time I had to make this hard call, we had two kids in college (one out-of-state, no less) and our oldest daughter had just gotten married a few months prior, so we were still recovering from some pretty hefty expenses while continuing to accrue more college debt. Our main bathroom had to be gutted and rebuilt at a cost of over $40,000, and maintenance on our house had gone through the roof with several other major repairs. I feel your pain and I know how much pressure you are under to just keep going on and on, but I also know you can only sustain this intensity and strain on your body for so long before it all falls apart. And when that happens, you won't be *any* good to anyone, including yourself or the family you are working so hard to support.

Why wait for things to fall apart (again) before doing something about it once and for all? This part of our process will help you focus on being mindful of *every*thing that impacts your health, from the way you wake up in the morning to what you think about on your drive to work and everything else that has kept you from getting out of this health nightmare.

Some of the most helpful things I have used for myself and with clients include:

- **Speed Bumps and Stop Signs.** I noticed that as I drove into work each morning, I'd get more and more anxious on my three-minute commute as my to-do list began taunting me before I even pulled into my parking place. I'd be in a hurry to just get in the building and start my day, but then I'd get into the parking lot and be super annoyed at the overly aggressive speed bumps that slowed my progress in getting where I needed to be. Then I thought about the purpose of those speed bumps – for us to pause and take a moment to evaluate a situation so we can move forward in the safest manner possible. I began to use speed bumps and stop signs as my reminder to notice my breath each time I encountered them. If it was shallow, I'd just make sure to take a deeper inhale and then I'd move on. It didn't add a moment to my commute. It didn't require me to write anything down. It simply gave me an opportunity to reground myself before doing the important work of teaching. How could that be a bad thing? Perhaps you have something you do throughout your day that you can use as your "speed bump" to remind you to "take a breath". Maybe each time you wash your hands or sit down in your car, you simply notice your breath and relax.

- **Write a cover page to your syllabus**, outlining appropriate times and methods for parents and students to contact you for work-related issues. (This is especially helpful if you are finding an expectation of 24/7 access to you by those you serve.)

- **Have a space that is exclusively yours**, whether it is a desk, office, or other location where you can work undisturbed. Put up a sign indicating when you don't want to be disturbed, and go ahead and close the door, put on noise-cancelling headphones, and do what you need to do.

- **Talk to your boss about reasonable expectations** and how you can meet them without having them snowball and become excessive. Before you have this conversation, though, take the time to outline your ideas so you know what your expectations will be. For example, how many after-school and evening activities are reasonable for you to supervise each week?

- **Enlist the help of others** by reaching out and asking for assistance. The more specific you can be with your requests (for example: I need someone to pass out programs from 6:30 to 7:30 at our concert on Thursday), the more likely you are to get people to help out and the easier it will be for everyone because expectations are clear. I have been incredibly blessed to have had the support of strong band booster parents and students during my teaching career. They can do amazing things if you are able to let go of the reigns and share responsibilities. Just be careful to ensure everyone is working to support the core values of your program and that everything everyone does is to support the kids you teach!

- **Start your mornings in a way that charges you up for the day.** Whoever thought high school jazz bands should meet at 6:30 every morning clearly never taught high school jazz band. That's a terrible idea! For most of my career, it took everything I had to drag my rear end out of bed at the last minute (5:15 a.m.) so I could hustle out the door by 5:59 and be at school in time to get the room opened and ready for the eighty kids who came in for the four jazz bands we had before school. By the time 6:30 rolled around, I was already frazzled ... until I reclaimed my mornings. I mentioned earlier that my new morning routine on school days starts at 3:30 a.m. I am literally ready to hop out of bed at that time because I know that time is all mine. I may get to share it with my husband while we have coffee, and I may spend time soaking in the hot tub, doing yoga, cooking breakfast, and meditating. I still leave the house at 5:59 in the morning, but when I do, I'm in a much calmer space and much more able to handle whatever comes later. I've come to treasure my quiet morning time more than staying under the covers and hitting snooze. Try a new morning routine for twenty-one days and notice how you feel when you start your day in a more focused way. (I'd recommend no electronic device use for at least the first hour.)

- **Reevaluate your work space** and make any changes that will be conducive to helping you work more efficiently. For me, that meant hiring a professional organizer. She and my husband and I spent a Saturday in my classroom, reevaluating how to use the room and my office to support my students' and my success. That meant getting rid of the stuff I "might need someday" and reorganizing my space so I could put things away when I wasn't using them. Reducing the clutter and being more visually organized helped me function much better, even after coming off my ADHD meds. It was freeing!

- **Plan meals and make time to eat them**. As teachers, we often skip meals, get very dehydrated, and end up eating junk food just to get instant (but not sustaining) energy. If you take the time to plan and take healthy meals to school, you're more likely to eat them – and then you will have sustainable energy to get you through your day!

- **Stay hydrated**. I found that the easiest way for me to stay hydrated was to get an electric tea kettle and keep hot water available during the day. By drinking eight to sixteen ounces of hot water with lemon and ginger each hour, I am able to stay hydrated. This makes a *huge* difference in my ability to think and focus. I also find that staying hydrated in this way has helped my skin clear up, I no longer get sinus infections, and all the headaches I used to get are gone. Hydration is pretty important – and it's cheap and easy to remedy, so *do it*! (I know that as teachers we never get to use the bathroom, but that's another issue!)

- **Incorporate time to upgrade yourself**. My mentor, Dr. Angela Lauria, shared how she came to the realization that self-care is really time when you are upgrading yourself to the next level. She's brilliant, so I am shamelessly stealing her fantastic advice not only in my personal life, but here in this book. Be sure you include time on a regular basis to address your needs and wants, from doctor appointments to massages and whatever else nurtures you so you can recharge and be ready for whatever comes next. You recharge your phone, computer, and every other device you own, so doesn't it make sense you need to recharge yourself?

- **Ask yourself, "Does this choice align with who I am?"** Any time you have to answer anything other than a resounding *yes*, then stop, take a deep breath, and decide if you really want to make that choice after all. Remember, it's okay to say no. Whether it's to another request for you to work overtime or to volunteer to be on another committee, ask yourself the question, "Does this choice align with who I am?" If the answer is no, then your response to the request should also be a no. You don't need to elaborate. You don't owe an explanation. Period.

- **Come up with a plan** that is sustainable. Talk to your boss, partner, students, cat, and whoever else is impacted by what you do and let them know how they can support you. Remember, in order for you to give them what they need, you need to be in a healthy place, so this kind of conversation can be win/win if handled properly. Think about strategies that allow you to be at your healthiest and how you fulfill your responsibilities best by working under those conditions.
- **Be aware**. Notice how you are feeling with each decision and adjust accordingly.

You are either succeeding or you are learning, so don't beat yourself up when things don't go the way you want them to. Use that as an opportunity to become aware of what not to do next time. It's this mindset that will make all the difference in your success or failure.

Action Plan:

Look at the suggestions above.

Which of the examples address the most pressing challenge in your work life?

Make a commitment to focus on one of these areas for the next twenty-one days.

1. What is the biggest challenge you face by not addressing this problem?

   _____

   _____

   _____

2. How will your life be different when this challenge is minimized?

   _____

   _____

   _____

3. What will you do *this week* to put this plan in motion?

   _____

   _____

   _____

4. Why is this important to address?

   _____

   _____

   _____

   _____

As you implement your plan of action, be sure to notice the impact not only on the specific area on which you are focusing, but the ripple effect on other areas of your life, too. You'll be amazed!

Chapter 11:

Some Practical Advice

*"Sometimes you don't realize your own strength until
you come face to face with your greatest weakness."*
– Susan Gale

Before you dive into the actual changes you are going to make, you must make a commitment to *why* and *how* you are making those changes. The *why* for me was I was physically too sick to go to work or do my other daily activities. I had no choice but to do the hard work of turning my life around or I would have kept getting worse. *How* I did it is what has now become the mPower Method.

When I was on a toxic cocktail of drugs in order to "function" (which I wasn't really doing very well in spite of all the pharmaceutical assistance), getting through my normal daily routine became impossible and I collapsed. I couldn't make one more decision. I was overwhelmed with responsibilities. I felt like my world was spinning out of control and the harder I worked at controlling everything, the more out-of-control things got. I was so busy being a people-pleaser to everyone else that I neglected my own needs, and by the time I'd been doing this for three decades, I was broken. I wanted another instant fix, but I had finally come to realize that the instant fixes I sought through traditional medicine really weren't working. Doing the same thing again was only going to get more of the same, and that would mean continuing in the downward spiral.

My friend Laurie had been diagnosed with stage IV ovarian cancer three years before I had my final breakdown. I watched her fight valiantly, and toward the end of her battle, I reflected on all of our conversations about our jobs, the stress of the responsibilities and demands, and raising a family and how that stress was showing up in our bodies through diseases. Unfortunately for Laurie, that disease had already rooted itself so deeply in her body that she never was able to be cancer free again.

She was very honest about how the stress affected her health and it scared the bejesus out of me. She reached out to me in spite of her own struggles, talking about alternative health care and other things I could do to get healthy, but it was too late for her. I loved Laurie like a sister, best friend, and confidante all in one and watching the cancer rob her of her quality of life, ability to be in her classroom, and opportunity to be a grandma while growing old with her husband made me realize that I had to honor her memory by sharing this message and technique with people like you so you can change the trajectory of your life before it's too late.

So here's where you have to trust the mPower Method, even when you feel like jumping ahead and quickly fixing everything at once. You've already tried it your way and it hasn't worked, so make the decision right now that you deserve to do this in a way that will change you at the core in a way that empowers you to *live* your life instead of just get through it.

The mPower Method was designed around the core principle of using mindfulness as the basis of everything. Once you establish the habit of being mindful, you apply it to every other aspect of your life. It becomes the core basis for decision-making, and it helps you make decisions that are in your best interest for getting to a better place in life and achieving your goals. It makes it easier to be successful with each step that follows once you have practiced being mindful and observing in a new way. Once you learn some mindfulness techniques, we will apply them in three other areas that impact your life the most: meals, movement, and music.

In essence, here's the plan:

MINDFULNESS PRACTICE THROUGH:
MEALS / MOVEMENT / MUSIC

Seriously, that's the whole plan. Think of mindfulness as the window through which we look at every other aspect of our lives. Mindfulness techniques will teach you to be in the present moment, observing rather than judging, shifting your attention from thinking to feeling, and when you understand how you *feel* when you do certain things, you make more decisions to do things that make you feel good. Make sense?

How do you make this happen? Where do you start? The dailyom.com outlines the **Five S's of Clearing** as slowing down, simplifying, sensing, surrendering, and self-care. This is where you begin. Our phones and computers need to be reset every so often or they slow down and stop working efficiently. You brush your teeth every day to clear the clutter from your mouth so you can start fresh. Doesn't it make sense that our brains, which have been "on" 24/7 since we made our entrance into the world, would also need an opportunity to reset? Of course it does. And now that you know better, you will do better.

This process creates awareness between your thoughts and actions and enables you to focus on managing your health problems and every other aspect of your life in a way that becomes your new foundation by inviting you to slow down and just observe what's going on in and around you. The steps we take might seem ridiculously small, but it's amazing how quickly these small steps accumulate and accelerate your progress.

I have a saying in my class: "We need to practice it until we can't get it wrong." Whether we are talking about learning to play a certain piece of music or how to eat in a way that provides us energy and helps us feel good, whenever we are developing a skill, we must practice it until we can't get it wrong. Then it becomes a habit. And when you nurture positive habits, your life changes drastically!

Christine E. Goodner says in her book *Beyond the Music Lesson: Habits of Successful Suzuki Families,* "Ten years from now, the fact that your child practiced on a random Monday in November is not a life-changing event. But who your child has become because they practiced daily *is.*" Replace the word *student* with *you* and you will understand the cumulative power of daily practice at a skill – Ten years from now, the fact that *you* practiced (or did something positive for yourself) on a random Monday in November is not a life-changing event. But who you become because you practiced daily *is*.

Think of this process like being on the freeway during rush hour. The roads are packed, making it impossible to get where you need to get without it being a hassle. Other people are in your way, the speed at which you are traveling is slower than a turtle's pace, and you're trying hard to zip around other people or find an alternate route. That's what your brain and body experience when you are constantly being stimulated by everything out there. It's like a traffic jam between all the connections of your nerves, muscles, and entire body. What you need to do now is get out of rush hour into a state where your oxygen and nutrients can travel where they're needed, where there's no interference from overstimulation to distract you at the cellular or larger level. That's essential if you are going to heal.

Slow Down: Take a breath and get centered.

Simplify: Get down to what is really important; most of what is bothersome is distracting but not the core issue.

Sense: Notice what you see, hear, taste, touch, and smell. This will help get you grounded and bring you into a space where you can respond rather than react to situations.

Surrender: Let go. It's freeing. You don't always have to be in control – and the more often you can practice this skill, the healthier you will be!

Self-Care: Or, as I mentioned earlier, "*upgrade yourself*" in ways that nourish your mind, body, and spirit. Everything from a haircut or pair of shoes to a walk on the beach or a retreat can be tools in keeping you your best.

Action Plan:

Commit to the *why, what,* and the *how* for this journey you are about to take.

1. *Why* do you need to invest in learning how to get healthy while working in a stressful career now?

   _____

   _____

   _____

   _____

   _____

2. How do you see the mPower Method supporting your efforts to reach your goals? List a specific technique from each step of the mPower Method you are committing to practicing for at least twenty-one days.

   Meals: _____

   Movement: _____

   Music: _____

   Mindfulness: _____

Come back to this chapter when you need to be reminded why you are on this journey and how you can get centered when things get overwhelming. Taking the time to step out of a situation, breathe, and notice how it's making your mind and body feel can save you immense stress, strain, and angst. Simply being aware leads you to make different choices. So take time every day, especially when you think you don't have time to, and literally breathe. Notice your environment. Engage all of your senses and take inventory of what you see, hear, taste, touch, and smell. That pulls you into the present moment, a place where clarity is within reach.

Chapter 12:

Put on Your Own Oxygen Mask First

*"Don't make someone go through
the same thing that almost ruined you.
Don't hurt people like that."*
– Anonymous

Y ou must take care of yourself. First. You can't give what you haven't got.

This is perhaps the hardest lesson of all, yet it is so important. Chances are you got where you are because you ran yourself ragged taking care of other people's needs. I bet you never said no to requests to be on one more committee, drive carpool, watch a friend's kids, and every other favor someone made of you, yet I'd also bet there's a good chance you never take the time to take care of your own needs. When was the last time you read a book for fun? Or went to a movie you wanted to see? Or pursued a creative endeavor that made you happy? Or did any one of a million things you want to do? I bet it's been a long time.

Well, that changes as of now. It's time to treat yourself with the same loving care that you give to other people. You must do this in order to demonstrate to the world how you'd like to be treated, because *ultimately other people will treat you the way you treat yourself.* I know this because I've lived it.

There was a time in my job where working twelve to fourteen-hour days was the norm, starting with a zero-period jazz band (at 6:30 every morning), filled with 200 to 300 students in six class periods, and at least one or two evening performances or events each week. It was grueling. But I just kept barreling through, taking on all the additional responsibilities that were being put on my plate either as requirements of my job or, in most cases, because the music program was growing so fast that there were a ton of additional opportunities for performances, trips, retreats, fundraisers, dances, and more.

What I didn't realize until many years later was that I was saying yes to everything that came my way, so I was essentially teaching other people that I was the go-to gal who could be counted on to do whatever needed to be done. I didn't respect myself enough to put up boundaries that would allow me to maintain a healthier balance between my professional and personal lives, and eventually it took its toll on my health.

Remember that example about putting on your own oxygen mask before helping others? This is where that analogy really comes in to play. It's time for you to take a good hard look at your self-care versus your care for others and decide if you are in a place where you have a good balance or if you need to make this a priority. (Hint: You probably are not doing very well in this category yet!)

Why is self-care / upgrade time such a critical component of your physical and mental health? Because in order for you to function at your peak, you need to meet the needs your body and mind have for rejuvenation, relaxation, and rebirth. If you are constantly putting out efforts toward other people and events but never taking time to refuel yourself, then you *will* run out of steam and it will manifest in your body as an illness, weight gain, acne, joint pain – you know the drill – again.

How do you begin to implement self-care as part of your daily routine when there are so many other things pulling your time and energy elsewhere? You make it a priority. And when you think it is selfish to put your own needs before someone else's needs, think about why you are holding this book. You're reading this because you've experienced repeated health issues and a big part of the problem that's led you to these health crises has been because you haven't taken care of yourself. That may include everything from skimping on sleep in order to catch up on housework to volunteering at your kid's school instead of going to yoga class or giving up your lunch period to help a student who's struggling.

While you certainly may enjoy many of the activities you do for other people, there are probably a lot of things you do that don't bring you joy or serve you.

I recommend you start by taking out your calendar and seeing what fills your days. Is there anything on your calendar within thirty days of today that is there solely because *you* want to do it, like a painting class or book club, a hike or coffee with a friend … or is there nothing there that qualifies? Your calendar undoubtedly has dozens of other entries indicating where and when you are doing everything from shuttling your kids to band practice or tutoring, going to PTA meetings, and more because you wouldn't dream of letting anyone else down. Now you are going to prioritize time for what *you* want to do, protecting it as fiercely as you do other people's events.

What you do for others is important and appreciated. If you want to continue to do good out there, you have to take care of yourself on a regular basis. We don't hesitate to write down important events in our calendar, yet when it comes time to prioritizing time for us, it's often done only as an afterthought, and then only if there's time and money that isn't needed for someone or something else.

That needs to change now.

You matter, and you need to put as much effort into setting time aside to nurture your mind and body as you do into everything else. If it feels selfish, think of it this way: When you are feeling fresh and at your best, you can give *so* much more to others. It's easier, more efficient, and less effort to accomplish everything you're trying to do if you are starting from a place that is centered and cared for.

What I found to be an important first step in self-care was setting boundaries. I absolutely love my job, and because I immersed myself in it for so many years, I showed others my enthusiasm. That enthusiasm was contagious, and before I knew it, the program was bursting at the seams with hundreds of students and their parents who shared my passion for making our music program the best it could possibly be.

I can't pinpoint the exact moment it happened, but at some point, my job took over my life, demanding more and more of my time and energy and leaving less for me to give to my family and myself. And the downward spiral began and never really stopped because I never took the time to reset and define some boundaries.

One of the most important lessons about self-care I learned came from a counselor I saw named Heidi. It was after I had hit that low point in the spring of 2017 and was working on ways to not only *get* healthy but *stay* healthy. I had sought the advice of various healthcare professionals, and I realized a mental health specialist was as important as my physician, naturopath, acupuncturist, and yoga instructors, so I found someone to help me establish a sustainable return-to-work routine.

Heidi began by giving me homework. (As a teacher, I'm usually the one assigning the homework, but now the tables were turned!) She told me to write the first page of my syllabus with information about *boundaries* for students and parents. I was terrified. I was certain that if I said it wasn't appropriate for them to come to my house to turn in homework (seriously, that happened), barge into my office without permission, or call my cell phone late at night to find out something they could have looked up online (or paid attention to in class when I announced it) that I would offend someone.

I resisted Heidi's instructions to be clear about office hours, appropriate ways to contact me, and other procedural activities she wanted me to outline in my syllabus. The more

I resisted, the more she helped me realize that *I had to model to others the way I expected to be treated.* If I continued to let people invade my family and personal time, then I was giving them permission to do so and it was my own fault that the ramifications were so hard on me. But if I respected myself enough to set up clear, professional, and family-friendly boundaries, then others could either respect that too, or their opinions would no longer matter. (I act all brave about that now, but I was pretty worried about being seen as letting down the kids and parents when I first expressed a need for people to respect my personal space.)

Guess what happened when I informed students and parents of these changes. People understood. They even said things like, "Good for you for reclaiming your space." They survived. And so did I. It was okay to advocate for my needs, and in doing so, I taught a very important life lesson to my students in the process. They were able to witness self-advocacy in a healthy situation in a way that may apply to them at some point in their lives.

Once I experienced the freedom and relief that came along with taking that first big step and setting boundaries, I realized I was actually becoming a much better teacher in the process. Since unnecessary work-related disruptions were no longer happening 'round the clock, I found myself far more focused on the students when I was present with them at school. It was as if we all knew we needed to use our time together more effectively because we weren't going to let things seep into other areas of our lives.

Setting boundaries is a necessary part of all healthy relationships, and by setting clear, fair, and firm (yet flexible when necessary) delineation between what is and what isn't acceptable behavior, you are empowering yourself and others to move forward with direction. Boundaries help people feel safe because they understand what to expect, so don't be surprised when you reap many positive benefits from this single step.

In addition to reestablishing appropriate boundaries, you can and must include self-care in your daily routine as well as on a regular basis in the bigger picture (think vacations, massage, etc.). If you don't, you will pay the price (which you already understand first-hand). When you become stressed or unhappy, it manifests itself in your body through illness, brain fog, or other physical or mental impairment. You won't be good to anyone, yourself included. If you miss the subtle clues like headaches, upset stomach, exhaustion, and the like, then your body will have to do something more drastic to get your attention, like develop a more serious illness because you didn't take care of what started as a minor illness, and that will put you right back where you were when you picked up this book.

When you take care of yourself, you become happier, healthier, and stronger. Others will see it and you'll begin to reap the benefits, and it won't take long until you understand that self-care gives you the strength, desire, and energy to reach the goals you have and live the life you dreamed. You deserve nothing less, and you can give yourself and others the best gift of all by taking care of you!

You teach other people how to treat you by how you treat yourself. If you are always putting other people's needs before your own, then you are teaching other people that

you don't value your own needs. Model respect for yourself and you will earn it in return. Neglecting yourself, not
taking care of everything from your health to your haircuts,
and allowing yourself to be last on your priority list shows
other people that your needs aren't important to you, so why
should they be important to them? There will be those who
resent you, especially at first, when you put up appropriate boundaries or refuse to get sucked into their drama, but
you'll find that letting go of that kind of toxic relationship in
the long run is healthier for you (and maybe even for them),
so be at peace with that decision and move on.

Action Plan:

As you think about how you are going to take care of
yourself moving forward, there are some other important
things to consider, such as:

- What kinds of boundaries do you need with colleagues? Friends? Family?
  - Do you want to maintain distinct separation
    between areas of your life such as work and
    family, or do you enjoy the overlap?

    _____

  - How will you communicate your expectations to
    others?

    _____

  - How will you model personal and professional
    boundaries?

    _____

    _____

    _____

- Tips:
  - Set your email to reply when you are out of the office so people won't expect immediate responses.
  - Post a "private" sign on your office or other space where others do not need to be.
  - Have a sign for your door that indicates "I'm working, please don't interrupt" so you don't have to keep being disturbed while trying to accomplish something.
  - Remember: you don't owe anyone an explanation if you choose not to do something.
- What are your non-negotiable priorities for *your* personal sanity?
  - What hobby are you going to make time to enjoy?

  _____

  _____

  - Why will you insist on writing your self-care events on your calendar? (Hint: If you don't approach your own desires with the same kind of commitment you do for everyone else, then you will stay stuck right where you are.)

  _____

  _____

  - What kind of movement will you do each day? What feels good in your body?

  _____

  _____

○ What will you incorporate into your *daily* routine that you will do for yourself *no matter what?* (This could be setting aside twenty minutes to read a book, FaceTime your best friend, enjoy a cup of tea, color, or do whatever your heart desires!)

_____

_____

_____

○ When will you do it? Get out your calendar. **For each of the next four weeks, write down three to four times you are going to engage in some kind of movement and another day you'll participate in an activity you do for your own enjoyment.** Hold yourself accountable for these appointments. And most of all, look forward to this time. *You* get to be your priority now!

Chapter 13:

It's Your Turn

*"Waking up to who you are requires letting go of
who you imagine yourself to be."*
– Alan Watts

O ne of my students, Emma, brought me a beautiful hand-painted mug last year. She had picked it because she said the colors (orange and blue) were the colors she associated with me, and because every day in every class, I always have a cup of tea nearby. It was the perfect gift. Since I drank tea every day, she knew it would get a lot of use, and she was right.

About a week after she gave it to me we were in class and I set it down on a music stand that had been tilted flat to function as a table. As you probably can guess, the music stand flipped and the mug went crashing to the floor. The sound was deafening. When I turned around I anticipated seeing a massive mess of ceramic chunks all over the place, but to my surprise, there were only two pieces of the mug on the floor, the mug itself and the handle. Nothing else was chipped or shattered. There had simply been a clean break separating the mug from the handle. I couldn't believe how everything else remained intact.

Once the handle came off, I could no longer use the mug for tea. It simply got too hot to hold when it had my tea in it, so I put it on my desk. I wasn't sure what I'd do with it, but without thinking I picked up a couple of loose pencils and pens that were scattered on my desk and put them in the mug. Suddenly the mug had a new function that I'd never have discovered had it not let go of its handle.

An object that had been created for the sole purpose of drinking hot beverages had been broken, gone through a transformation, and emerged with a new purpose. It was no longer limited to being a tea cup. Instead, it could hold pens and pencils. Or it could be used to drink cold beverages. Or I could use it as a vase. Or for candy. Or for any of a dozen other purposes now. I never would have noticed all its potential if the handle had remained intact because in my mind, the handle clearly defined it as a cup for hot beverages. Removing the handle opened up so many more potential uses for the mug.

The same is true for you. You are probably gripping on to some things that hold you back or limit your progress, even if those things aren't bringing you joy or no longer serve a purpose for you. Getting out of the rut you're in requires looking at the "handles" (which can include people, habits, mindsets, fears, and more) that are holding you back and letting them break off so new possibilities can arise.

Think about your personal situation. You're obviously on a journey of self-awareness and are committed to making progress, and in order to make that progress, you have to identify where you are in the six stages of personal change and figure out what you need next. Look at the stages and see if you can identify where you are today. The stages are:

1. **Being stuck**
   ◦ Not caring if you change.
   ◦ Not even sure what you want.
   ◦ Not sure how you'd get what you don't even know you want.
   ◦ Might not even care to change things because it seems like too much work.
   ◦ Depression lives here.

2. **First doubts**
   ◦ What do I want to do?
   ◦ What do I have to do?
   ◦ I can't do that...*can I?*
   ◦ Do I care enough to get out of this rut?

3. **Self-questioning**
   ◦ What am I meant to do?
   ◦ What's my purpose?
   ◦ Am I reaching my potential?
   ◦ What is my potential?
   ◦ What do I see myself doing in five years? Ten years?
   ◦ Who am I to be special?
   ◦ Am I good enough?
   ◦ Am I worthy?

4. **Seeking change**
   - My life isn't working the way I need it to.
   - I know there's something better for me.
   - I feel like there's something I'm called to do.
   - I don't know what it is, but I know I have to make a change in my life.
   - I need to have a purpose.

5. **Finding change**
   - I'm seeking information about a hobby, going back to school, taking a vacation, or something else that's new.
   - I found something that helps me be more physically active.
   - I completed a health assessment and am trying a new habit that will help me reach my goals.
   - I am actively doing something that makes me feel whole (fills my soul, gives me purpose).

6. **Reintegration**
   - I have created new habits that have led me to additional healthy choices.
   - I see the changes I've been seeking to make happening in me and the universe seems to be bringing me more of the things I need to keep this momentum going.
   - I like how I feel and will do whatever it takes to continue on this path.

Being stuck can and will happen to you. There will be many obstacles that get in your way of making progress. You will probably be your biggest obstacle, because change is hard. It's scary. But *not* changing is even scarier, so when you get that urge to throw it all in, stop, take a deep breath, and take stock of what you are feeling. Acknowledge the challenge. Feel crappy for a minute or two. You can't change what you don't acknowledge.

The Soul of Leadership reminds us that in order to solve a problem, we must first *acknowledge* it and *feel* the impact of it. Once you've owned it, the next step is to *feel* the solution. Imagine how you will feel when you've solved the problem, then actually feel that way now.

Become the person who has solved the problem and you're halfway there. That was how this book and my coaching practice were born. I saw the problem with my personal health and the health of my colleagues who were suffering a myriad of physical and mental stress from the demands of their jobs. Once I *acknowledged* the severity of the problem and watched my best friend die of cancer while other friends and I continued to get unhealthier, I *felt* the devastating impact of continuing down this high-speed path to destruction in my declining health. And then I began to be open to what being healthy would *feel* like, and that's when my behaviors began to align with what I needed to do to achieve those goals. Every time I question if I'm on the right track, I come back to asking myself *how I feel* when I make a particular choice (to eat a certain food or to spend time on social media) and then I make the decision about what to do based on how I want to feel. It's liberating!

It will be hard sometimes. The rest of the world will be going along at its typical crazy speed while you are trying to get a handle on things. It won't stop so you can regroup and get grounded, but you *can* make progress toward healing, even when it feels impossible.

In my personal life and when I'm working with clients and students, I have found that when a problem really and sincerely needs to be solved, that's the time to double down on the support in order to be successful. It's during these major events or challenges when getting the one-on-one guidance is of utmost importance. During my band classes, for example, I can address the needs of the ensemble, helping students fix things that impact the group, but when I get the opportunity to coach someone one-on-one, we can dig in to root-cause and focus on building skills or setting up new habits that are specific to their short- and long-term goals.

When I am working with students who are mastering an instrument and have a performance coming up, they'll often turn to weekly one-on-one lessons (private coaching) so they get specific and timely feedback, enabling them to improve their skills not only for the short-term concert, but also develop those skills they will continue to use as long as they play an instrument.

The same goes for you. Now that you've realized you've got to shake things up and make significant changes if your life is going to get better, you're ready to take it to the next level. You've already figured out what *doesn't* work. You've wasted time, money, and energy – not to mention a lot of hope – on short-term fixes that were more like Band-Aids and not genuine healing. You've invested in doctors, books, diet plans, and dozens of other quick remedies, yet you're reading this book because you still haven't found the right path for your journey to wellness.

If you're like me, it's overwhelming to think about where to start. There are doctors, naturopaths, traditional medical practices, alternative medicine, drugs, psychotherapy, diets, exercise plans, food intolerances to consider, and the list goes on. Not knowing where to begin can be debilitating and a roadblock that you just can't overcome in order to move forward.

When the same old routine is no longer effective and trying to figure this out on your own hasn't worked, doesn't it make sense that this is the time to double up on your support, too? Don't you deserve to finally get the results you desperately need? You have so much more you want to do in your career and life, yet your health isn't supporting those goals. Finding the support where you have someone holding you accountable is key.

My middle daughter is brilliant. She was talking about why people should see life coaches and counselors. Since she's a musician and actress, she made the connection between people seeking one-on-one coaching to help them understand themselves and having private instructions to learn to play an instrument. She is so right. By enlisting the help of experts in the field in which we are struggling, we get that personalized feedback that helps us set, reach, and surpass the goals and dreams we have for ourselves.

When I finally came to the realization that I couldn't solve my medical problems by continuing to treat each symptom independently and that I needed to explore other options, I reached out to every resource I could for support. I started by reading everything I could get my hands on. Then I went online and gathered more information. I visited different kinds of healers. I tried alternative therapies. And guess what – when

I did different things, I got different results! Not all of the results were good, but by bringing my awareness to how each kind of treatment plan made me feel, I could move forward making decisions that supported feeling good. In other words, *I* had a lot more control over my destiny than I ever realized.

I couldn't have been nearly as successful in reclaiming my health as I've been had I not been receptive to working with other people. I had learned what *didn't* work, so it was time to learn what *did* work. I needed their help, and I'm so glad I accepted it.

As you reclaim your health, I encourage you to reach out and use whatever resources you need in order to maximize your success.

FREE RESOURCES

Facebook support groups

In-person support groups

Mental health counseling through work (often provided at no charge through HR)

Friends

Colleagues

Professional associations

Online resources

Walking or other activities you enjoy

Community music groups

Sports teams

LOW COST SUPPORT

Self-care (massage / hair / nails)

Self-help books

Yoga or other gentle movement

PRICELESS SUPPORT– Your better tomorrow starts today!

One-on-one coaching – mPoweredEducator.com is a list of my resources, tips, and coaching offerings

Retreats

Classes

Now that you *know* better, you can *do* better. You just have to be willing to do the work, and the way to be most efficient and effective in your endeavors is to reach out and find the help you need. At the end of this book there's a chapter of some of the resources I found to be invaluable in my search for healing. What started as a journey to get my physical health in better shape has ultimately accomplished so much more because I was willing to dig deep, feel the pain, and realize I didn't want to feel that way anymore.

My wish for you is that you find the help you need to conquer the chronic stress, exhaustion, and sickness that is inherent with your career and family lives being so full. You have given to others to the point that you have nothing left to give for yourself or anyone else. But now you are holding a book in your hands that has a plan to help you turn things around immediately. Use this book and the plan in it to make big changes. It will be hard work, but isn't everything that's meaningful worth working for?

When you were learning to play an instrument, you probably had books you used to help you build skills. This book is just like the Hanon Exercises for Piano and Arban's Brass

Method books – it has the steps you need to learn in order to make progress toward your goals.

Perhaps you learned just fine by using the books and practicing on your own. Or maybe you took private lessons, where you had a teacher work one-on-one with you to help you work through the books in a more effective way that got you results more quickly and helped them be permanent. You can approach your health in the same way. You can use this book as your guide. Set aside time to read each chapter, do the action plans, and hold yourself accountable.

Getting healthier, regaining energy, being less stressed, and returning to work with vigor and fresh enthusiasm is possible – and *you can do it.* Growth is painful. Change is hard. But nothing is as painful as staying stuck somewhere you don't belong. What will it be for you?

Action Plan:

If you are ready to invest in permanent positive changes, reach out to me at <u>Lesley@mPoweredEducator.com</u> for a free consultation to see if we'd be a good fit to work together. We'll design an individual plan that addresses *your* goals and circumstances so you will be able to find permanent positive changes that allow you to conquer the chronic exhaustion, stress, and sickness once and for all!

> *"If you don't make the time to work on creating the life you want, you're eventually going to be forced to spend a LOT of time dealing with a life you don't want."*
>
> – Kevin Ngo

Powerful Resources You Should Use

O nce I began this transformation in earnest, I sought every possible resource in my effort to understand *why* I felt so crappy and exhausted. Helpful advice from my family doctor, naturopath, acupuncturist, yoga teachers and nutritionist, combined with valuable content from countless books, magazines, videos, and classes taught me how much control I actually have in how I feel. By focusing on what I eat and how I care for my mind and body, by practicing daily mindfulness, I have learned how to positively optimize my health and life/work balance, and I hope you will too. Here are additional resources to help your on your own journey of personal growth and transformational change.

Super Woman Rx by Tasneem Bhatia, MD (Dr. Taz)

Grain Brain by David Perlmutter, MD

The Bulletproof Diet by Dave Asprey

The Secret by Rhonda Byrne

The Soul of Leadership by Deepak Chopra

Eat Bacon, Don't Jog: Get Strong. Get Lean. No Bull___. by Grant Petersen

Head Strong by Dave Asprey

The Influential Mind by Tali Sharot

Brain Maker by David Perlmutter, MD

Miracle Mindset by JJ Virgin

Inheritance: How Our Genes Change Our Lives and Our Lives Change Our Genes by Sharon Moalem, MD, PhD

Happiness the Mindful Way: A Practical Guide by Ken A. Verni, Psy. D.

Mindfulness: A Practical Guide by Tessa Watt

Mindfulness in Action: Making Friends with Yourself through Meditation and Everyday Awareness by Chogyam Trungpa

Steal like an Artist: 10 Things Nobody Told You About Being Creative by Austin Kleon

Brain Bytes: Quick Answers to Quirky Questions about the Brain by Eric Chudler and Lise Johnson

The Music Lesson: A Spiritual Search for Growth through Music by Victor L. Wooten

Quieting the Monkey Mind: How to Meditate with Music by Dudley Evenson and Dean Evenson MS

The Seven Spiritual Laws of Yoga by Deepak Chopra, MD, and David Simon, MD

The Brain: The Story of You by David Eagleman

Lessons with Love: Tales of Teaching and Learning in a Small-Town High School by Marianne Love

Happy Teachers Change the World by Thich Nhat Hanh and Katherine Weare

Thinking Just Hurts the Team: Find Happiness and Ignite Your Full Potential by Taking the Principles of Yoga to the Workplace by Salisa R. Roberts

The Second Circle: Using Positive Energy for Success in Every Situation by Patsy Rodenburg

Acknowledgments

There are many individuals and groups of people who have been instrumental (band joke) in making not only this book but my life's work possible. At the top of that list is my family, starting with the love of my life and soul mate, George, who has been a rock by my side for over thirty years. I can't imagine sharing this adventure with anyone else but him and our three daughters, Kelly (and Brandon Block), Meagan, and Nicole. Right beside them in this journey have been my parents, Bruce and Jo Caldwell, who have been my biggest advocates, cheerleaders, and mentors. Encouragement from my brother, Steve Caldwell, and sister, Traci Owens, has helped me make it through whatever obstacles have come my way. And a special shout-out to my nieces, Angela and Kristina Owens, for their makeup and photography skills.

Through all the health issues I've experienced, I'm grateful to have had some remarkable doctors who have been by my side, including Dr. Mark Anderson, Dr. Kate Kass, Heidi Howard, Dr. James Pautz, Dr. Miriam Mendelsohn, Dr. Youl Park, Dr. James Alberts, and Dr. Aric Christal.

I've been humbled by the support of the incredible Henry M. Jackson High School staff, with a special shout-out to Dave Peters, Michelle Renee, Blythe Young, Shaun Monaghan, Setchin Tower, Kevin Hall, Drew Baddeley, Melanie West, Craig Schell, Brian Marshall, David Lamoreux, Storm Benjamin, Gary (and Sue) Martin, Willie Sandygren, Kenneth Walker, Superintendent Gary Cohn, Georgia Lundquist, Keith Corning, Shelly Henderson, Teresa Jacobs, Curt Cheever, our School Board, and the Everett Public Schools for supporting the arts in education.

The words "thank you" are insufficient to express my gratitude to the countless students and their families with whom I've had the privilege of working over the past three-plus decades. The love, support, and camaraderie felt in our band family has sustained me when I've been in some unhealthy places, and for that I am eternally grateful. Thank you to Jared Kerber, Lili Martinez and Emma Raker for encouraging me and giving me the courage to take what I learned through my personal health journey and share it in a mindfulness practice with my students. You inspire me!

Carrie and Bruce Wallace and Morgan Ward, owners of Yoga in the Center in Mill Creek, Washington, and their phenomenal instructors: Andrea McLaughlin, Lyndsey Huntington, Mara Critchett, Leslie Robbins, Judi McGee, Debra Meyer, Janiece Collopy, Liz Abendroth, Kate Towell, and Christina Cavoretto. Kim (Frederickson) Parker has introduced the healing powers of Tibetan sound bowls to me and to my students. Andrea McLaughlin's assistance with learning about nutrition was incredibly helpful and a key to my continued success.

So many people have directly or indirectly had a huge impact on who I've become as a music educator. They include Kwane McNeal, Tom Morgan, Casey Whitson, Chelsey Caldwell Eisenhower, Caitlyn Malarkey, Nyla Fritz, Janet and Mike Hitt, Vanessa Gerads, Sarah Fowler, Dr. Laurie Cappello, Kirk Marcy, Gerry Marsh, Steve Fissell, Dave Golden, Terry Cheshire, Walter Cano, Daniel Halligan, Sue Piatt, Nicole Whiteley, Megan Vinther, Patrick West, Ben Lee, Frank DeMiero, Marianna Smith, Kelly Clingan, Dr. Tim Lautzenheiser, Peter Tiboris, Allen Vizzutti, Nancy Ditmer, Michael Butera, Frank DeMiero, Tam Osborn, Kelly Caldwell, Jim Rice, Jim Kovach, Danny Helseth, Larry Gookin, Mark Lane, Dr. Brett Mitchell, Keith Brown, Frank Batagglia, and Dr. Brad McDavid.

The information I learned from reading books by Dave Asprey, Dr. Tasneem Bhatia, and Dr. David Perlmutter has been a game-changer. Read their books!

When things got tough, it would have been easy to quit, but there are a lot of young women out there who are carrying the torch in music education, and I want to see them continue to forge ahead and thrive in this amazing career. This is for *you*: Charlotte Reese, Suzie Reese, Ainsley (Leavitt) Holz, Monica Weber, Esprit (Sager) Cummings, Amy Stevenson, Janelle Arenz Beal and all the rest of you!

Thank you to Danielle Barnum of https://www.inspire-bydanielle.com/ for sharing her superpower of her art of photography and helping her clients step into their power through pictures.

To those who encouraged me to write this book and the friends and family who have been by my side for a very long time, I love you guys! My fabulous in-laws, George and Pat Moffat; Barbara Sleeper; Janie McDavid; Deanne Bodyfelt; Kelly and Guy Block; Sharon Jackson; Carol Kovach; and Michelle Warnke.

Of course, *none* of this would have been possible without the structure, guidance, and support of the incredible team at The Author's Way, led by none other than Dr. Angela Lauria. Her amazing staff includes Sharon Pope, Ramses Rodriguez, Cheyenne Giesecke, Bethany Davis, Ora North, Jennifer Stimson, Natasa Smirnov, Tara Kosowski, and Trevor McCray. The team at The Author Incubator has also asked me to acknowledge the Morgan James Publishing Team: David Hancock, CEO & Founder; my Author Relations Manager, Gayle West; and special thanks to Jim Howard, Bethany Marshall, and Nickcole Watkins.

THANK YOU

As a thank you for reading this book, I've got a couple of bonuses for you!

BONUS: You are invited to **join the private "I Love My Job, but It's Killing Me" Facebook page.** It's exclusively for people who have gotten this book and want to have a place to interact with each other and with me through content and Q&A opportunities.

On this page, I'll personally answer questions and I'll share pointers that you can use to get on the road to a healthier you more quickly and with more sustainable results than if you try to do this on your own.

By joining this community of people, you'll find tons of support amongst others who are on this journey. You can share your successes and challenges, and you can ask me for input, too!

Take advantage of this limited time offer by going to mPoweredEducator.com/VIP. Simply enter your email address and I'll send you the link to this page. Can't wait to meet you there.

BONUS: If you answered true to more than ten of the questions on the Mojo Meter, you can set up a **free**, no-obligation **coaching call with me**.

I can help you identify the ways you can use the mPower Method to jump-start *and* sustain you on your health journey, with tips that will help you transform and regain your health and energy quicker than you imagined was possible. Go to https://mpowerededucator.com/book-an-appointment/ to sign up for your private 45-minute call with me to go over your personal results and plan.

The hardest part is booking the call. Once you do that, I've got your back! Let's do this.

About the Author

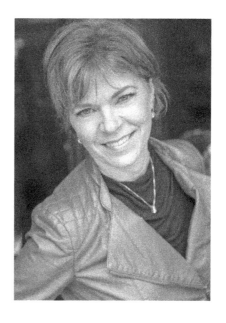

Now in her fourth decade as a high school band director, Lesley Moffat has worked with thousands of people, helping them not only achieve musical goals (including repeated performances at Carnegie Hall, Disney Theme Parks, Royal Caribbean cruise ships, and competitions and festivals all over the US and Canada), but also teaching them how to develop the long-term life skills they need to be successful in the world.

Following multiple serious illnesses and surgeries, Lesley had to completely transform her life at the age of fifty-one to prevent her health from continuing to decline. Using her body as a laboratory while desperately searching for cures from doctor after doctor, she became fed up with traditional band-aid approaches to treating symptoms, finding she just ended up sick again and again.

Now healthier than she was in her thirties, Lesley's ready to share her secrets of success with a larger audience. A teacher at heart, she has designed a program to help women who find themselves chronically sick due to excess stress and exhaustion to reclaim their health so they can reclaim their lives. In the same way that she's designed lessons to engage *every* kind of learner for the thirty-plus years she's been a teacher, she is able to create individualized plans that meet the specific goals of each client on their path to a healthier and happier life.

Lesley has been a presenter at the National Association for Music Education (NAfME) and WMEA Conferences, served on the board for the Mount Pilchuck Music Educators Association, and is an adjudicator and guest conductor in the Pacific Northwest.

Lesley lives in the same Seattle suburb where she's taught for most of her career, developing relationships with students and their families as their teacher and also as a fellow member of the same community.

After completing her undergraduate degree at Indiana University, she returned to her roots and moved back to the Pacific Northwest, where she and her husband, George, raised their three daughters, all of whom were students in her high school band program. Fun fact: Lesley, George, all three of their daughters, and Lesley's dad have performed at Carnegie Hall.

CPSIA information can be obtained
at www.ICGtesting.com
Printed in the USA
LVHW090524300122
709553LV00004B/440

9 781642 796216